The
DIVINE THREE MANUAL

Books by Jay Gutierrez & Faye Gutierrez

The Divine Three Manual: How to Heal Yourself Safely
and Simply Using Earth's Natural Resources
The Hormesis Effect: The Miraculous Healing Power of
Radioactive Stones (Jane G. Goldberg, Ph.D.,
with Jay Gutierrez)

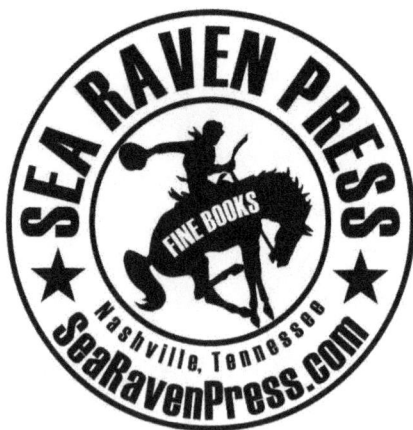

THE
DIVINE THREE
MANUAL

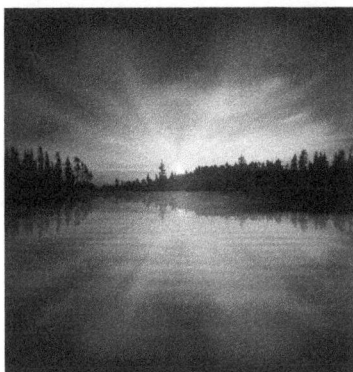

HOW TO HEAL YOURSELF SAFELY AND SIMPLY
USING EARTH'S NATURAL RESOURCES

JAY GUTIERREZ AND FAYE GUTIERREZ

ILLUSTRATED

Lochlainn Seabrook, Editor

SEA RAVEN PRESS, NASHVILLE, TENNESSEE, USA

THE DIVINE THREE MANUAL

Published by
Sea Raven Press, LLC, founded 1995
SeaRavenPress.com

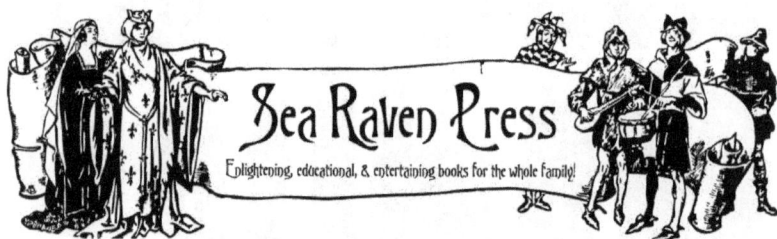

Sea Raven Press
Enlightening, educational, & entertaining books for the whole family!

First Sea Raven Press Paperback Edition: October 2014
ISBN: 978-0-9913779-7-8
Library of Congress Control Number: 2014946412
This book is also available as an ebook.

The Divine Three Manual: How to Heal Yourself Safely and Simply Using Earth's Natural Resources, by Jay Gutierrez and Faye Gutierrez. Edited by Lochlainn Seabrook. Includes an index.

Front and back cover design and art, book design, layout, and interior art by Lochlainn Seabrook. Typography: Sea Raven Press Book Design. All images, graphic design, graphic art, and illustrations © Sea Raven Press. Cover image: © Lochlainn Seabrook.

PROUDLY WRITTEN, DESIGNED, AND PUBLISHED IN THE UNITED STATES OF AMERICA.

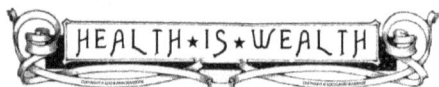

HEALTH ★ IS ★ WEALTH

CONTENTS

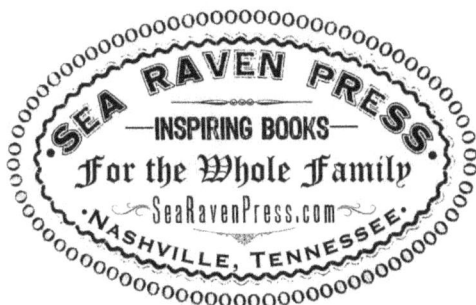

SEA RAVEN PRESS
—INSPIRING BOOKS—
For the Whole Family
SeaRavenPress.com
NASHVILLE, TENNESSEE

DISCLAIMER

This book is for educational and informational purposes only and may not be construed as medical advice. It is not intended to replace the services of a physician, nor does it constitute a doctor-patient relationship. You should not use the information in this book for diagnosing or treating a medical or health condition. Always consult a physician in all matters relating to your health, and particularly in respect to any symptoms that may require diagnosis or medical attention. Any action on your part in response to the information provided in this book is at your own discretion.

The Authors

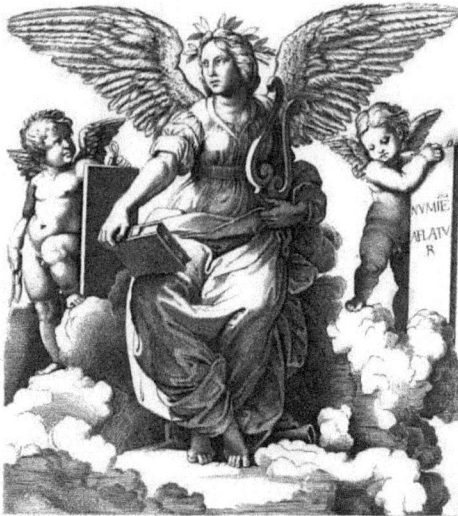

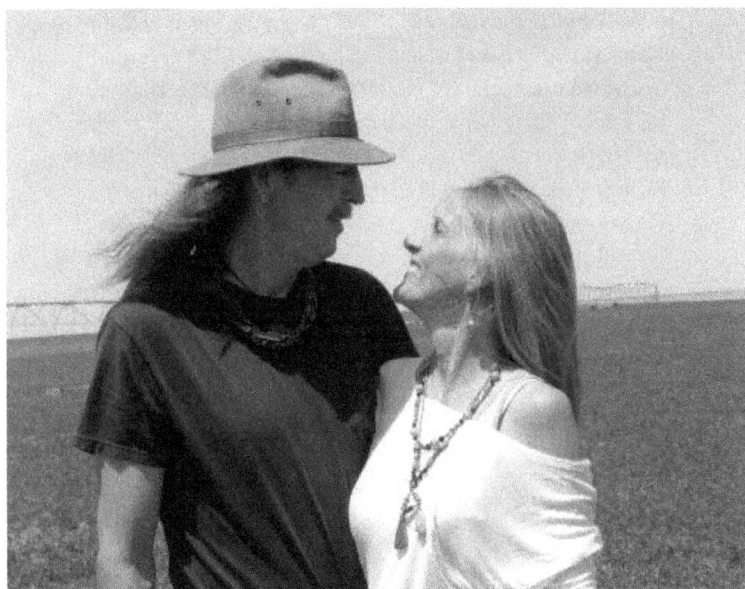

Jay and Faye Gutierrez.

Dedication

OUR FRIEND AURA

At a time when we really needed someone special to come into our circle and help with a unique situation requiring the 24/7 care of an ALS client, God sent us Aura! She arrived with everything she owned and seemed to know she was there to offer her services. That was the beginning of a relationship with Aura and it has grown stronger over the years. We have never met someone that was this caring and loving, who abundantly is always there to serve His will. Aura has had much experience in aiding others, as she showed us during her time here in Pritchett, Colorado. She was instrumental in the preparation of our wellness manual, and helped us put into place many tools we use to this day. She will always have a place here with us—but it is very hard to keep an Angel in one place. The world is a much better place with Aura here to teach us compassion, humility, love, and how to serve Him to the best of our ability.

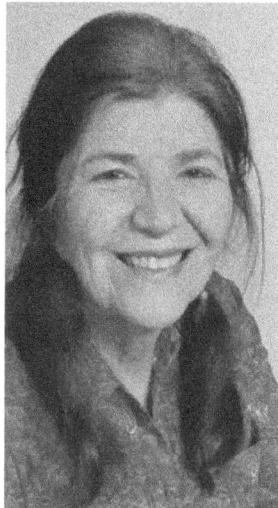

INTRODUCTION

HAVE YOU EVER NOTICED HOW uniquely rich the experience is, when you are witnessing someone who is so totally "in their element" and living their life with such a deep commitment to service, they seem like a magnet for creating extraordinary events and breakthrough situations? Jay Gutierrez is one of these remarkable people.

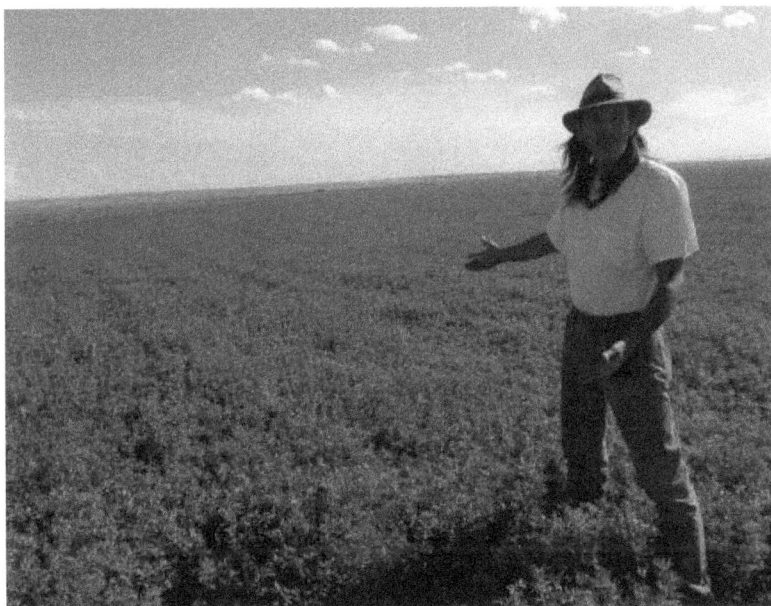

Jay has a checkered past. After growing up on a farm and finishing high school in Berthoud, Colorado, he joined the Air Force. Acing the entrance test, he was encouraged to choose whatever field of service within the Air Force that he wanted. Opening the service book to a random page, he looked at the picture and said, "I'll do that. I'll be a jet engine mechanic." After six years of service and war time experience, he joined the Army.

With more commendations than he is comfortable talking about, and an honorable discharge, he settled into his career as a helicopter mechanic.

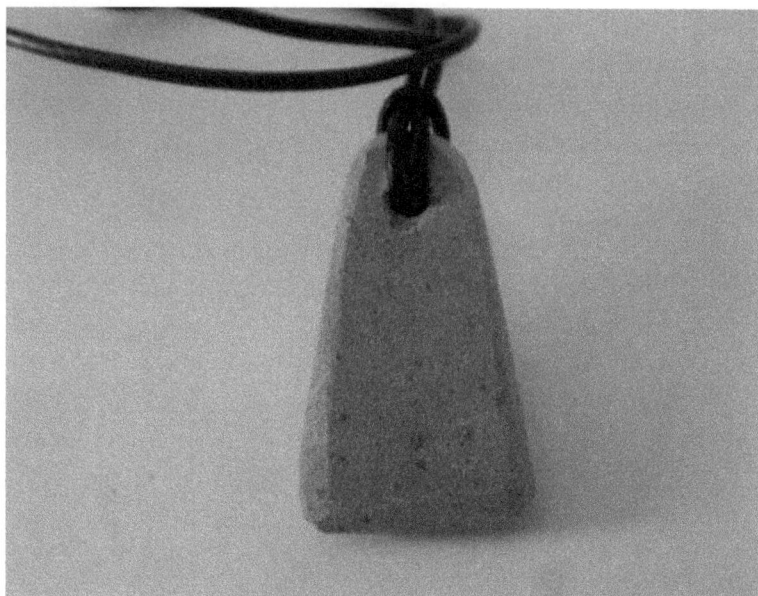

Our popular book, *The Hormesis Effect: The Miraculous Healing Power of Radioactive Stones* (which Jay co-authored with award-winning New York psychoanalyst and renowned alternative medicine expert Jane G. Goldberg, Ph.D.), offers a poignant perspective:

> . . . in the midst of gathering the stones, giving away the stones, and compiling anecdotal evidence of the value of the stones, a very fortuitous thing happened to Jay. He went to prison for a year. He willingly became the fall-guy for an elaborate scheme of his superiors that involved re-positioning (some would call it "stealing") helicopters. But Jay made good use of his time in prison: he devoted

himself to doing research to find out why slightly radioactive stones would have the effect of healing people with such a wide array of afflictions. And in his research, he came across a scientific and medical concept that was to change . . . the lives of the countless "patients" he has worked with, restoring them back to health, saving their lives.[1]

Through those experiences, Jay began opening his heart and mind to the kind of help and wisdom which only comes from listening to the Stillness and having personal conversations with God. In Pritchett, Colorado, and beyond, Jay Gutierrez also has had help from far more than just a few friends.

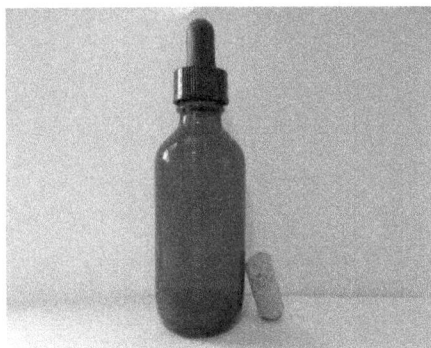

One is an astute Executive Officer who keeps everyone grounded and focused on service. Faye Gutierrez, Jay's wife, experienced life changing results from Jay's amazingly magical rocks. She is now a stunning and articulate presenter of radiation hormesis frequencies. And Faye's son, Daniel Cox, is a trained, highly skilled Wellness Instructor with Night Hawk Minerals, whose service included a tenure within the healing center, Carpenter's Grace, of Scott and Liz Carpenter in Lafayette, Oregon.

Another is a holistic family medical doctor of 35 years in practice,

---

1. Goldberg, Jane G., and Jay Gutierrez. *The Hormesis Effect: The Miraculous Healing Power of Radioactive Stones.* Nashville, TN: Sea Raven Press, 2014.

who supports Jay's program as Medical Director for Night Hawk Minerals. Dr. Raphael d'Angelo's philosophy is to uncover the root causes of problems while helping each patient set high expectations for ongoing wellness and health. His patients are generally seeking natural, complementary and alternative options while saving traditional medical approaches for instances when they are most needed.

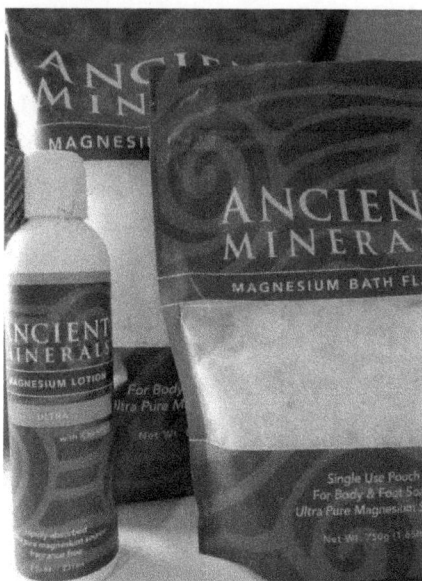

Jay and Dr. d'Angelo met in the spring of 2006. Jay came to his office with his radiation stones and testimonials. The doctor was skeptical, but after trying it on himself and several of his patients, he became convinced that Jay's radiation hormesis works. They soon developed a genuine shared respect which evolved into a mutual intention to join forces and expand their professional services to help save lives.

Dr. d'Angelo's wife, Nancy, supports her husband's interests from her own company providing optimal and completely trustworthy therapeutic quality essential oils, hydrolats, hydrosols, and expressed oils from impeccable sources around the world. Nancy is a Certified Clinical Aromatherapist. Her company is Julia Rose Botanicals.

Additional support has come from a divinely guided connection with Walt and Kathy Merriman in Alabama. With 25 years of research and continuous endeavors to "get it right," they offer mineral waters that are truly Divine by adding water soluble, naturally ionized, angstrom sized minerals that our bodies were designed to use. These minerals are truly "organic" in nature; they are 10,000 times smaller than colloidal minerals and are 100 percent effective in the bodies of humans and animals. Because they are 100 percent absorbed by the cells, they leave no heavy metal residues in the body. Now at last minerals are able to perform their intended functions—and the results to date are truly amazing. Walt says, "The body will heal itself. It's not magic. Let us show you how." This he has done!

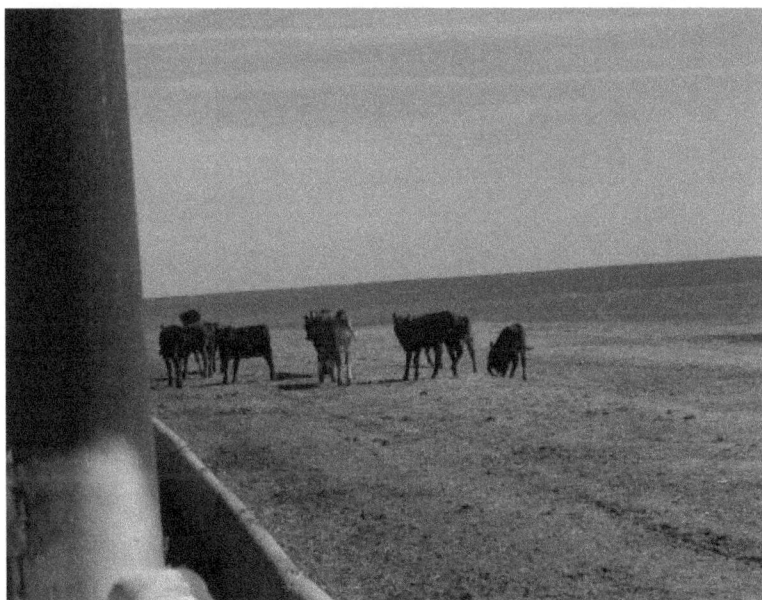

Above and beyond the professional liaison with these extraordinary healers, what is very important to Jay is that on the other side of the veil, there are angels and Archangels, guides and spirit friends, as well as the Son of God, who undoubtedly sit in counsel as Jay converses with God about his clients and their particular needed protocols for healing.

From this spiritual bond, the inspired triangle of extraordinary healers, and precious relationships with clients, *The Divine Three Protocol* emerged. Here is the compelling story as Jay tells it.

> Of course we knew from irrefutable evidence that our radiation hormesis stones were saving lives. Yet, as the years passed and we gained so many more experiences with clients, we realized there was a bigger picture and more pieces to the puzzle of healing diseases.

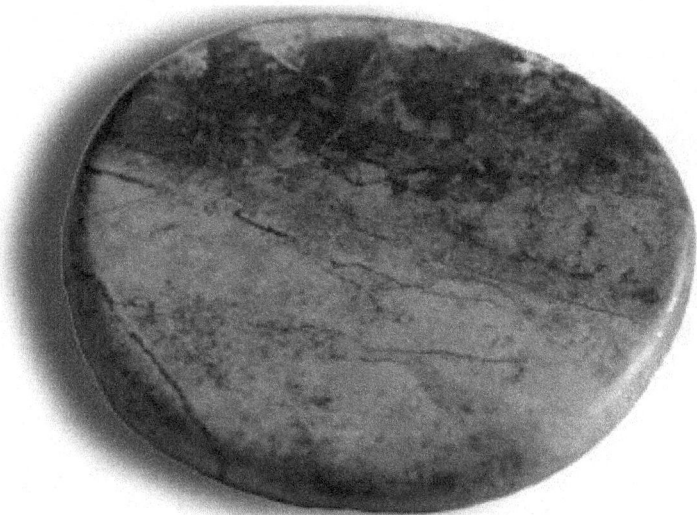

> It began when Dr. Hammed Ibraheem, from Nigeria, Africa, heard my talk in 2008 at the New York Life Expo. He understood what I was saying and how important the connection was to his work. Even though he is the leading parasitologist in the world, I did not get the connection between the

extensive damage the parasites do to the tissues, the toxic waste the parasites excrete and the overwhelming, explosive supply of yeast/candida that shows up in an attempt to eat the dead tissue, excreting more mycotoxins, which actually creates more food for the candida. That's your cancer!

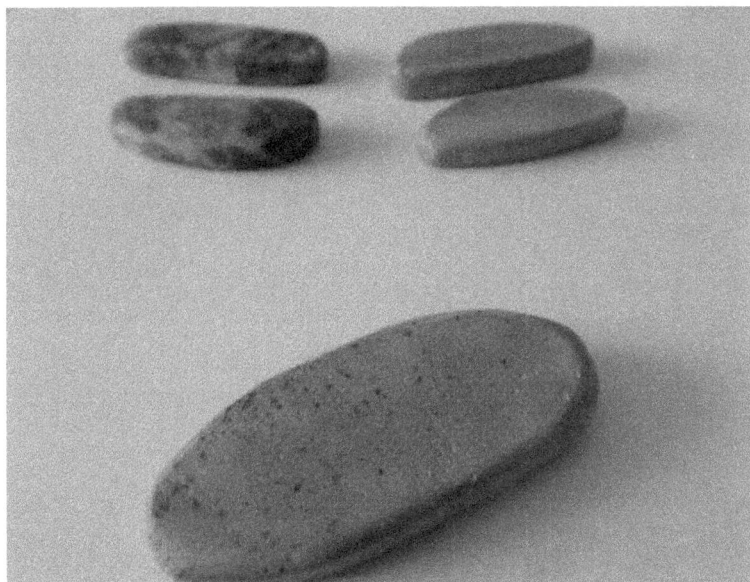

I didn't connect the dots until we met and worked with Kelly in 2009. She was a beautiful mom with two very young daughters. After seven years of all kinds of treatments, and visits to healers all over the country, she finally died from cancer which had spread from her liver to the spine and then all over her body. She told me about the number of times she was tested for parasites and was told the tests were negative. As she described her symptoms and the painful internal movement she felt going across her body, I suspected parasites.

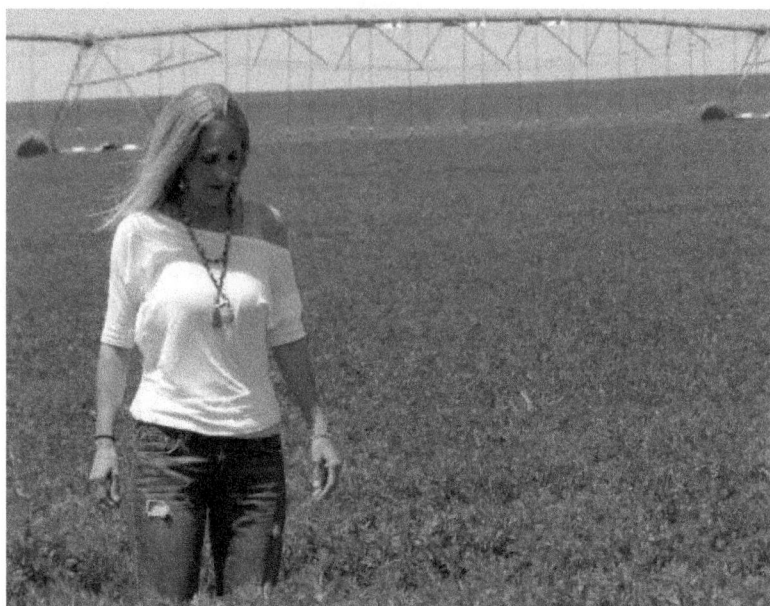

Several months before she died, we sent her stool
sample to Dr. Ibraheem in Nigeria. The tests
showed that she was full of parasites. The remedies
were over $3000.00. We raised money on the
internet to help her get them. By the time they
arrived, she was too weak to do any of the cleanses
and her immune system was completely
compromised from her mainstream medical
treatments. So we all watched in heartbreak as she
died. Thanks to Kelly, we learned beyond a
shadow of doubt, that parasite identification and
specific parasite remedies are a critical piece of the
healing puzzle.

That's when I found out that Dr. d'Angelo is also
licensed as a parasitologist and agreed to join forces
with me. At the beginning of 2011, he took over

our parasite testing program, which has now become the third part of The Divine Three Protocol.

At the beginning of 2012, we pulled out our files and matched diseases in clients and their symptoms with the exact same symptoms caused by specific parasites which he had identified, especially in patients with leukemia and breast cancer.

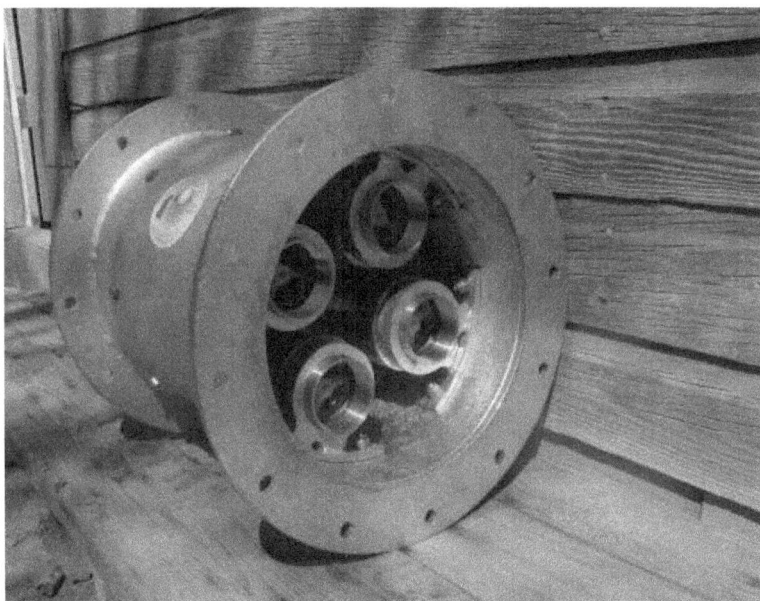

Ascaris-type round worms, were found in people with breast cancer, and men with prostate cancer. Going by "what we see," one of the most destructive creatures out there are round worms. Breasts and prostate glands are made up of a similar type of tissue. Round worms are attracted to that type of tissue. By taking time to go through our files together, "light bulbs" of understanding went off about how parasites are frequently the underlying cause of degenerative inflammatory diseases that will not be stopped until the cause is removed.

So how did the second part of The Divine Three Protocol fit into this picture? It happened on one of our long road trips across the country in early 2011. After losing Kelly, I had been praying hard to connect the dots to the bigger picture of why some people were doing all that we knew to provide for their healing and still losing the battle. When Faye and I were introduced to a bottle of angstrom sized mineral water in Minnesota, we immediately suspected we had a piece of the healing puzzle in our hands.

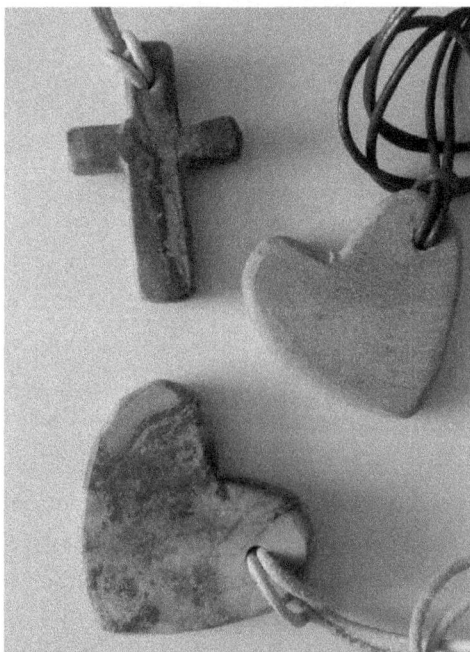

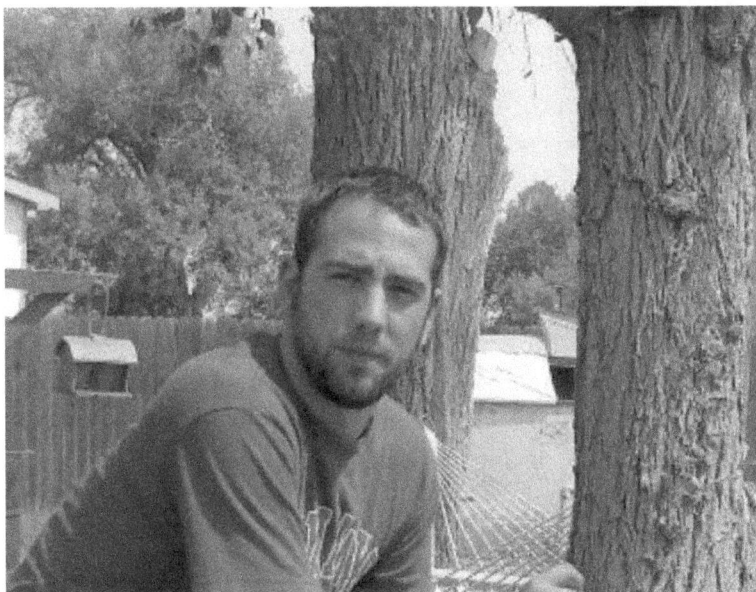

Daniel Cox.

We did the leg work to discover Walt and Kathy and their Water Divine company in Alabama. With an invitation to come down, in the spring of 2011, we all spent a couple of days together and I learned about the Amish people in the area Walt had been working with for fifteen years. While we were together, a client contacted us having a heart rhythm problem. Walt discovered that her heart pressure medication had a diuretic in it. He knew that meant she was losing potassium which is essential to keep the heart beating in rhythm. When her doctor was consulted, the doctor agreed to balance her medication with potassium. We've learned since that she's doing great!

We saw first hand the wisdom they had acquired in their years of studying how these minerals, vitamins

and enzymes operate synergistically in the body to
help the body deal with deterioration, disease and
illness by providing it with the elements it needs in
a 100 percent usable form. As we witnessed the
extraordinary success Walt and Kathy were
facilitating, and the success rate Water Divine
minerals, vitamins and enzymes were having, we all
began to explore the possibility that God was
calling us together to "hold healing hands" to
integrate the essential elements of radiation
hormesis frequencies, and mineral waters as two of
the three distinctive parts of The Divine Three
Protocol."

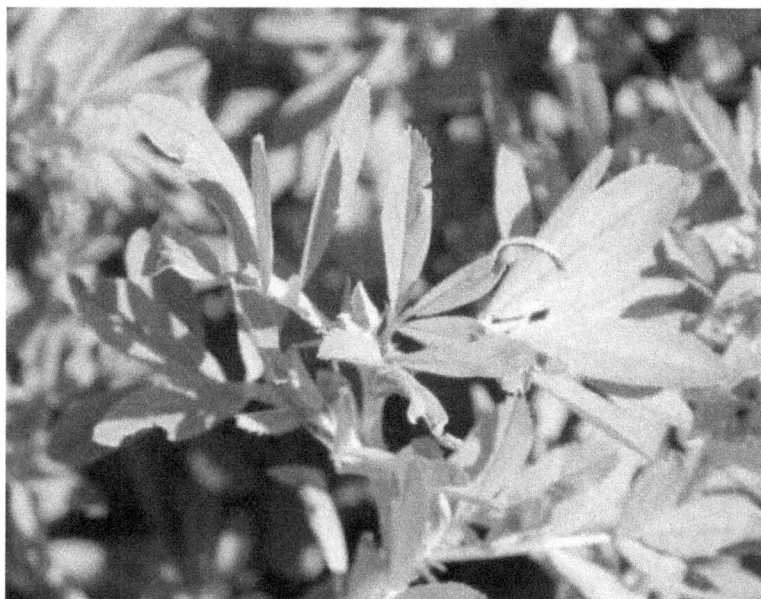

So here we are in the summer of 2014, and because
we are all now working with the synergistic power
of The Divine Three Protocol, the present and
future opportunities to provide complete healings

from degenerative diseases for people and animals
are brighter and brighter.

Chapter 1 of this manual is intended to give you more information
and reasons to pay attention to the expertise and wisdom being
garnered by these gallant, life saving, game changing heroes.

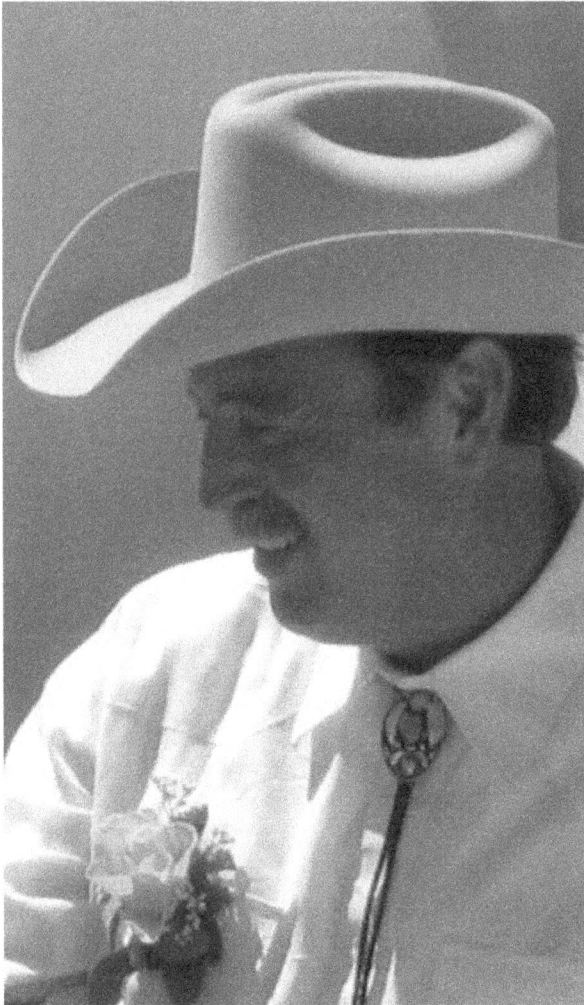

Jay Gutierrez.

The

DIVINE THREE MANUAL

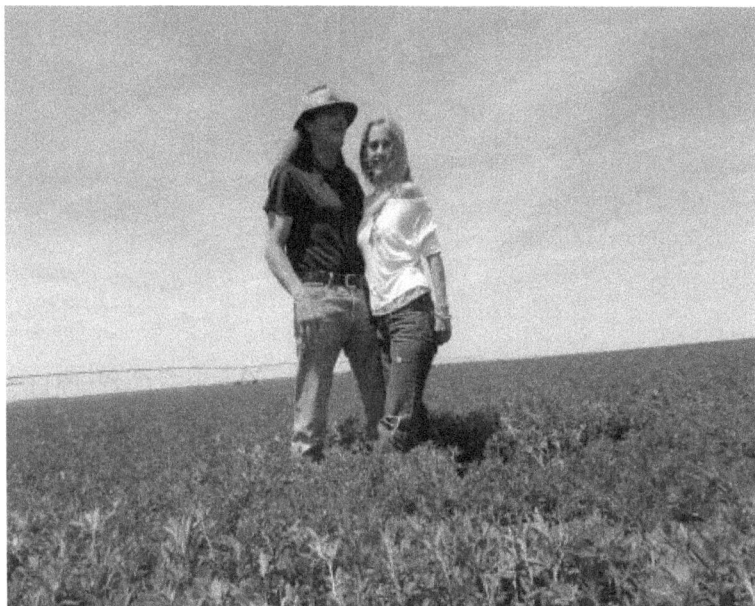

HOW TO HEAL YOURSELF SAFELY AND SIMPLY
USING EARTH'S NATURAL RESOURCES

1

THE DIVINE THREE PROTOCOL MUSKETEERS: WHO ARE THESE GALLANT, LIFE-SAVING, GAME CHANGING HEROES?

THERE ARE TIMES WHEN LIFE seems rewarding, beyond measure. Especially if you, or someone you love, is facing a life threatening disease, you may decide that getting to know these three couples is one of those times. This section of the manual will give you a larger glimpse into who they are, and why they have joined together to be of greater service to you.

It's easy to think of Jay Gutierrez as the "Master Mind" of the group because, in his disarming enthusiasm and humbleness, he often reports on the messages he has received from God, whom he honors and reveres as his Master in guiding him to a greater understanding of how to engage and support the team—his extraordinarily capable Executive Officer-wife, Faye, the Night Hawk Minerals Medical Director, Dr. d'Angelo and Assistant/wife, Nancy, and the Merriman's, Walt and Kathy, in Alabama, as they provide The Divine Three Protocol to people who come from all over the world.

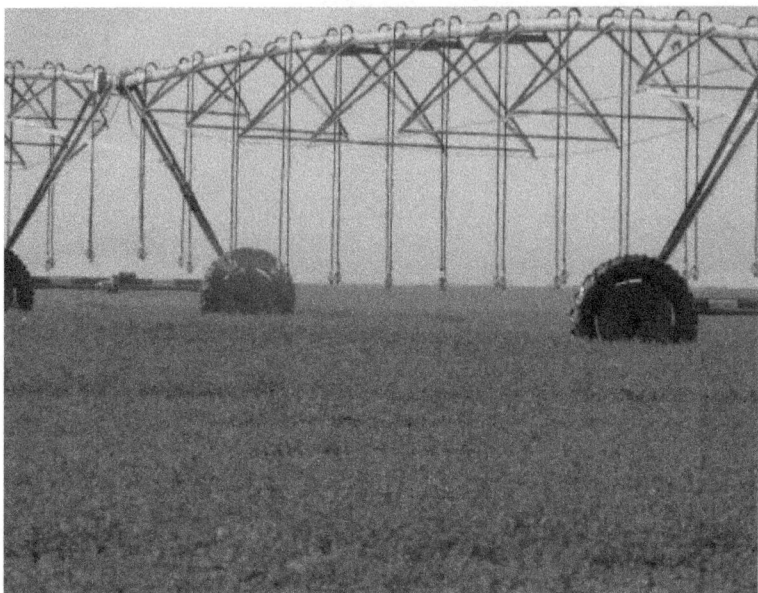

The best way this writer could think of, to give you some greater insight into discovering who these special healers are, was to invite these empowered wives to talk about their husbands and tell us their stories—who they know their husbands to be, the history of their work, and why it is so important to the world.

FAYE GUTIERREZ'S STORY:

> I met Jay in 2005. In 2006, I joined the staff where he worked in a helicopter company in Denver, Colorado. At that point, I had always had sinus problems and allergies, and was just not really feeling good over all and not being able to give 100 percent. So one day, I went down to his office to take a flight with him to see how his work is performed out in the field. By doing that, I got some one-on-one time with Jay. He gave me my very first stone, which I don't use now, because it's

my very first one! So he told me some of his history. He talked about the qualities of the stones, and the calls he was getting. I thought it was really interesting.

Jay quickly and easily became my medical mentor as I slowly revealed what my physical issues were. At first, I was scheduled to do a colonoscopy and I cancelled the appointment. He also knew I was dealing with some eye issues. He did not know I was dealing with some breast issues, intestinal issues, hemorrhoids, yeast infections; the list was very long. And so one at a time, I would ask him about them. I didn't find out until later that I was the very first person he witnessed as the toxins came out right through my eyes. All the infections and poisons in my body seemed to exit right through my eyes.

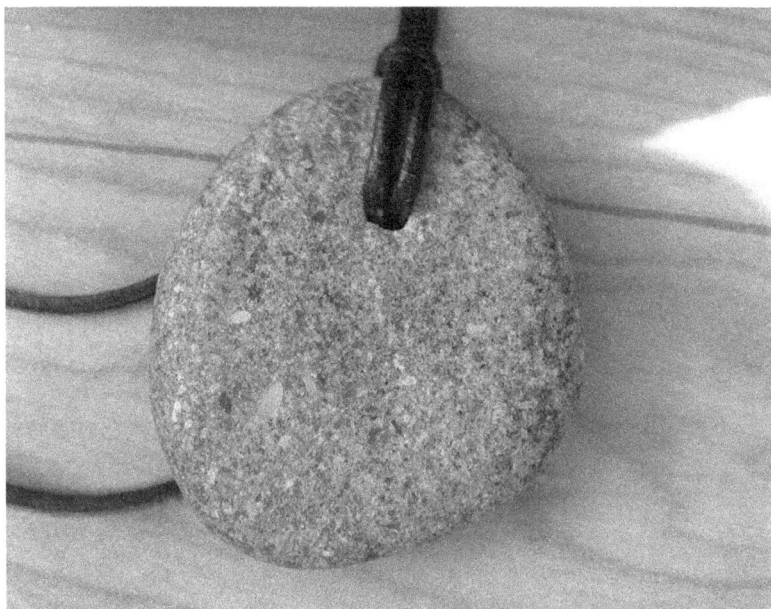

So I told him, "You're on to something here pal, and whatever you want me to do, I'll lend a hand on weekends and help you out." With so much going on, I finally got up the courage to go see Jay again and say, "Jay, I've got this pain going from my armpit right up to my nipple and my breast seems to be tender and leaking. His eyes lit up and he already knew from his studies what was going on, because he was already working with similar problems. So again, he gives me another rock and it's a hot rock. The first stones he gave me were the Green Stones for my eyes.

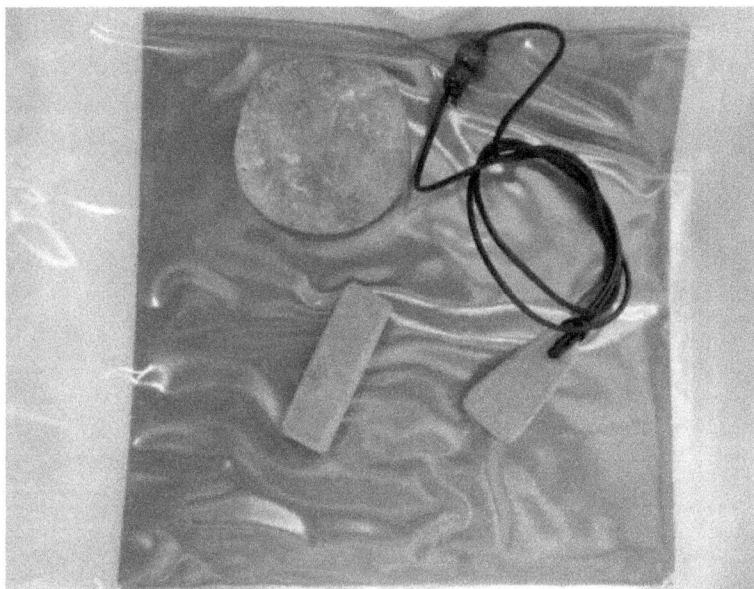

He said, "Put that right there. Wear it every night, *every* night with your mudpack." So I did everything he told me to do. I had no idea what the problem was, and I will never know because it is gone. This was 2007. It all happened so fast. I met him in 2005. Then I went to work for the helicopter company in 2006. We started addressing my issues in 2006 and 2007.

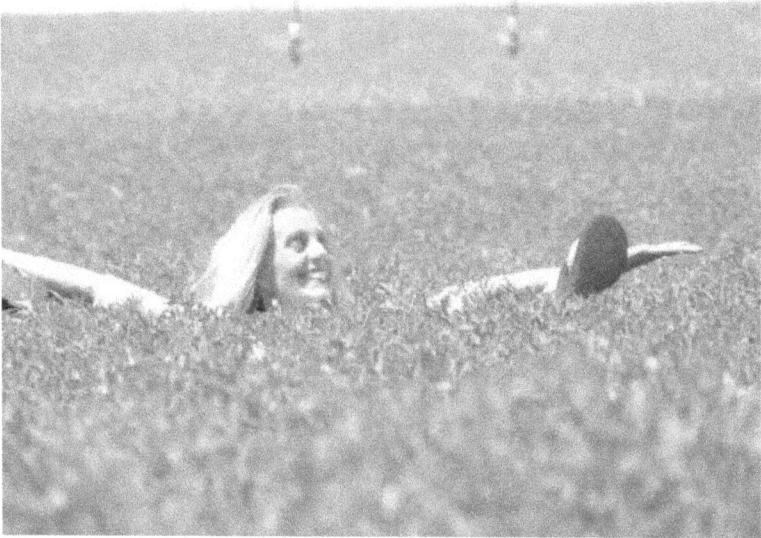

As we went further, Jay came to me one day and asked if I wanted to go to a lecture with him. I had tickets to a concert but gave them away to go and work with Jay. After two lectures, it took 30 days for us to decide to be business partners. A very special friend, Carol Thomas, helped us open the doors of our company, Night Hawk Minerals, in The Mineral Palace in the center of Pritchett, Colorado. Carol created the first brochure. She was the one who said to me, "I think there's a man there who adores you. I think you ought to look into it." Jay walked away from me one day and turning back said, "You know you're going to be mine, don't ya?"

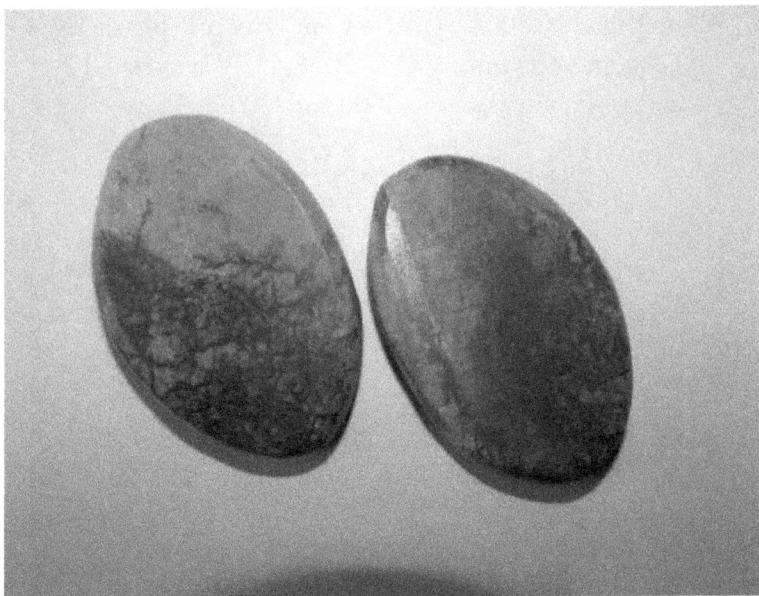

To be honest, I didn't see him coming. I prayed to God for a lot of years about who and what I needed and God transformed Jay right before my eyes. You can see his pictures on the website. Go all the way back to 2008 to look at pictures of Jay then and now. I tell him all the time, "We are getting younger!" He looks younger now than he did then! From all that we were learning from our clients, Jay began to believe it was the radiation hormesis frequencies that were doing the job of healing, and the frequencies are very much about anti-aging. He laughed and said, "Look at me!"

We talk a lot these days about the life-giving frequencies of the "hot rocks." The energy of the frequencies is so healing. We are learning more and more about how positive energy puts out a healing frequency and how negative energy stops healing frequencies. My son Dan will say, "You can imprint that water with your thoughts." And he's right!

Now, we're busy filling the Mineral Palace with positive healing frequencies. To start with, on September 25, 2008, we took an old hotel in Pritchett, Colorado and transformed it from the first day of October to opening the doors on November 15, the same year. We wanted to welcome people to feel like they were in their home away from home. The Mineral Palace is very spiritual. It has its own really unique abilities. So we're where we are supposed to be. We've made it our home and between the Mineral Palace, a Volunteer Servers cottage close by, and guest quarters in our Rock House, we welcome people as guests to come and heal their bodies, minds, and spirits.

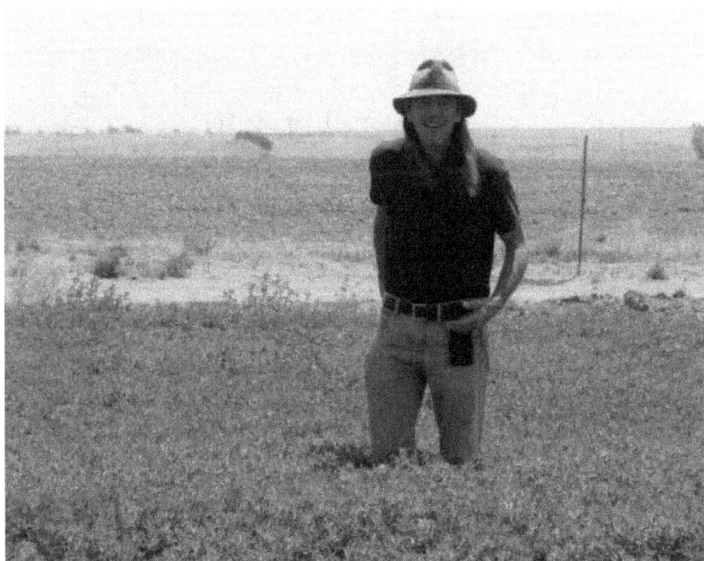

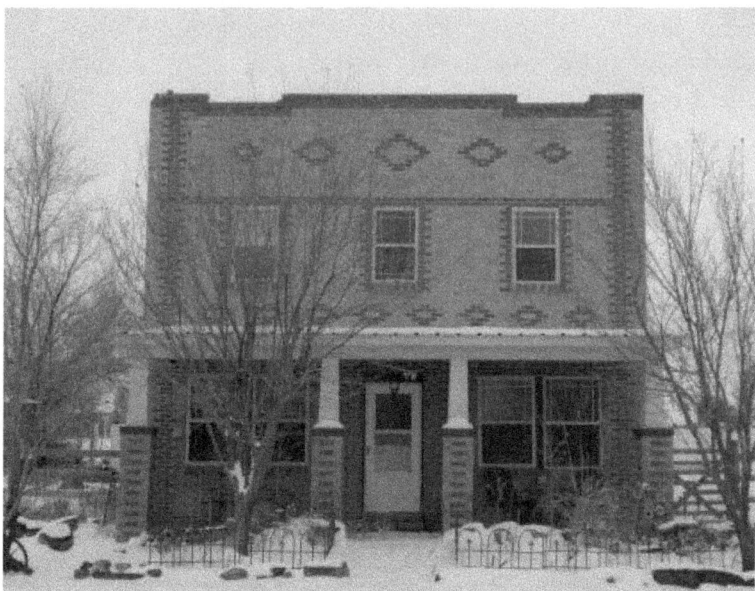

Levi's Bed and Breakfast, where our Night Hawk Minerals' guests stay.

Jay is truly my knight in shining armor. We had always worked well together, so we quit our jobs with insurance and benefits and went to work in a field that no one recognizes, because we get rewarded by helping people every single day. It's a "hard sell" because people don't get it. Jay is a very quiet, always thinking kind of guy. The stones brought us together. And, even on the tough days, we get a great reward of opening the mind of just one person to reconsider their options.

There are weeks when the phone does not stop ringing. Still, we're sitting in heaven on earth because our mission is to support people with information that can save their lives and ask them to take some time to do their own research.

Jay understands that what he has to offer is not new. From the 1800's and 1900's to the early 1940's, radiation hormesis, as a healing modality, is very old. The government used the radiation fallout from the nuclear bombs to scare people away from it. And, from working with our thousands of clients, our journey has now taken us to understand the synergistic healing impact of The Divine Three Protocol.

What we are all saying to people is this: we have uncovered what is out there, available to you naturally. You don't have to necessarily do anything else. It is most important to first take the time to listen to yourself, do your own research, and follow your own mind and heart to and through your healing process.

And every day I say to Jay, "God is great!"

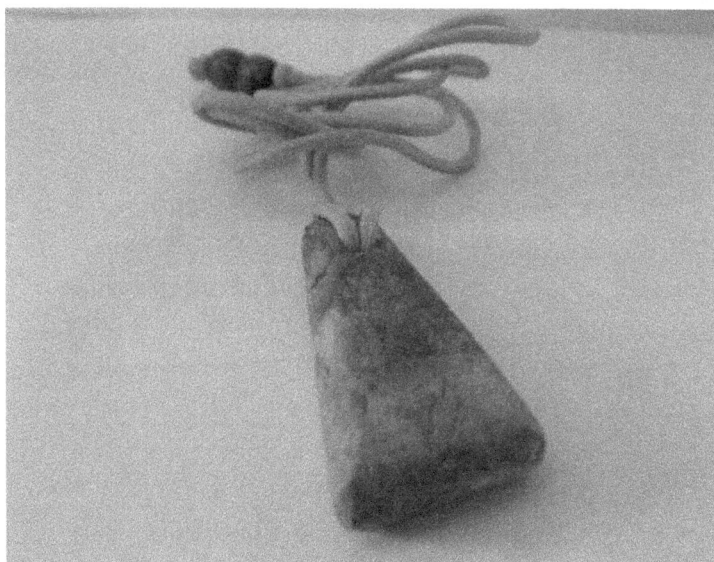

KATHY MERRIMAN'S STORY

Kathy and Walt Merriman began their journey together over thirty-three years ago. Kathy says:

> I still love him. I still like him. And I can still ride in the car with him for eight hours and enjoy it. *And* I think he would say the same about me. Really, I think I've been more difficult to live with. He's real easy.

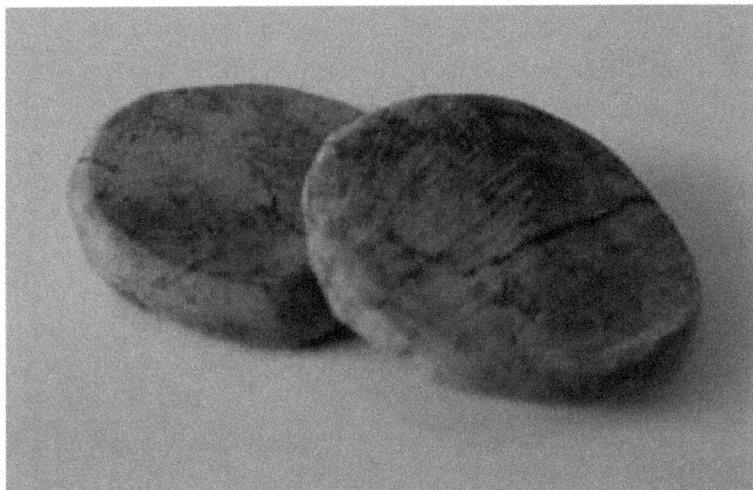

> Our family and our customers mean the world to us. We have five kids. Our children work here. We're a family who really cares about each other and we are very happy in what we do. Our customers love us. They genuinely appreciate what we do for them. Customers don't keep coming back unless your products are worthy.

When Kathy was asked, "Why should the world know about your husband's work?" her enthusiasm rose. She said:

Because it is life altering, completely life-changing. He has information that you cannot find out at the local drug store. His information comes from over twenty years of research, and his knowledge is far superior to anything else on the market. Where ever he goes, people listen.

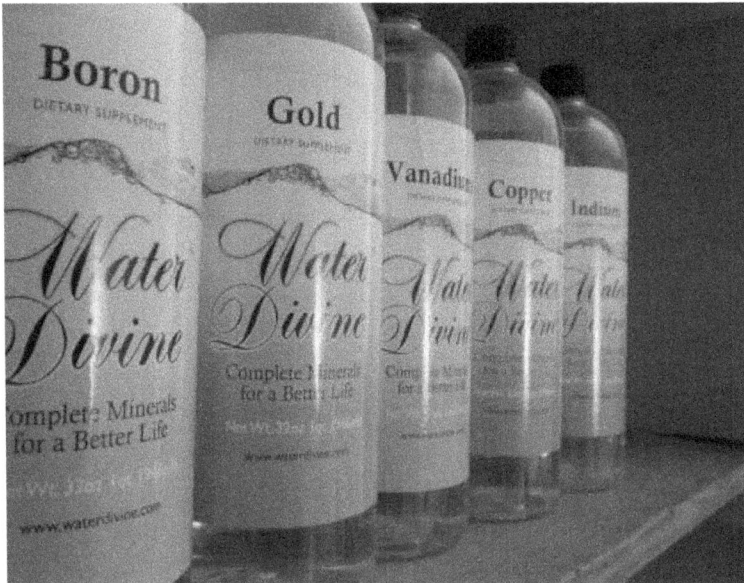

It was easy to hear in her voice, the great admiration and deep respect Kathy has for her extreme researcher husband. Kathy says he has the ambition to retrain America with the understanding that all disease is indeed a nutritional deficiency.

Walt states:

> Understanding the cause of a disease is far greater than suppressing the symptoms. The body will heal itself, but it's not magic and real nutrition is required.

Kathy continues:

> Walt has a strong passion for helping people get well, and his uncanny ability to zero in on an individual's nutritional inadequacies comes from his vast research, gathering and retention of uncommon knowledge.
>
> From 2000 - 2004, he served as a national director in an alternative healthcare organization which grew from a small service company to a publicly traded leader in the alternative healthcare arena, while he was the lead instructor at all of the national events. Today, he's one of the nation's leading and recognized wellness consultants, hosting his own television show, each weekday, called "Your Health Matters" with Walt Merriman. He is much sought after as a public speaker, radio host and lecturer.
>
> His message is simple. The great people of America have been oppressed. The oppression and abuse appears to come from the pharmaceutical industry. His mission is to uncover the truth and bring it to the American people.

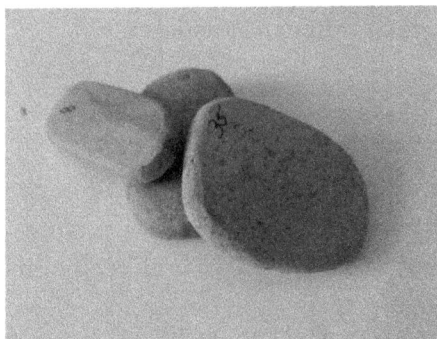

One thing Kathy says to Walt every day is: "I praise God for what He has given me." She spoke with a lot of humility and went on to say:

> He's given me my life with Walt, and my 5 children, 7 grandchildren, and 2 on the way. We have a great life and a great business. We get to help people live a better life every day.

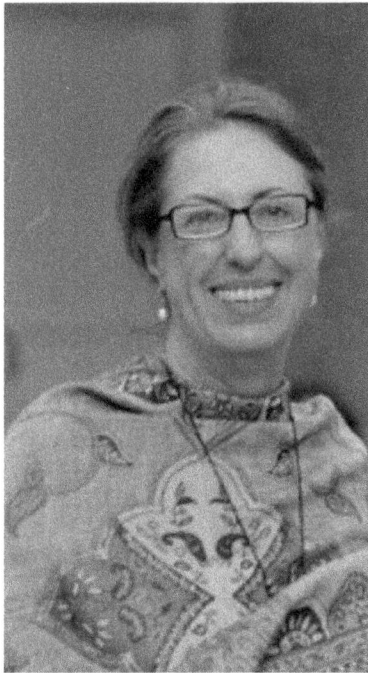

NANCY D'ANGELO'S STORY

Nancy d'Angelo became aware of her husband, Dr. Raphael d'Angelo in the late 90's. Having already raised a beautiful family, at the time they met, life was presenting her with the necessity to claim her independence as she moved forward. She was working in a flower shop in Denver, Colorado, learning much about the essences of plants and flowers, and especially the "life blood" of "her new babies," called essential oils. Nancy worked as a florist for 18 years, and has worked toward learning nutrition and herbology all of her life. As a well respected herbologist, today Nancy operates her own company, Julia Rose Botanicals as a certified clinical aromatherapist.

Nancy d'Angelo.

While Dr. d'Angelo and Nancy were becoming more aware of each other in the late-90's, during that time she learned many things about the energetics of flowers. Nancy says:

> There are very few people who can look at a beautiful bouquet and not want to smell it, or walk into a room with a gorgeous arrangement and not be drawn toward the fragrance. Most often, it will change the person's mood. When you change the mood, you change the behavior as a direct result.

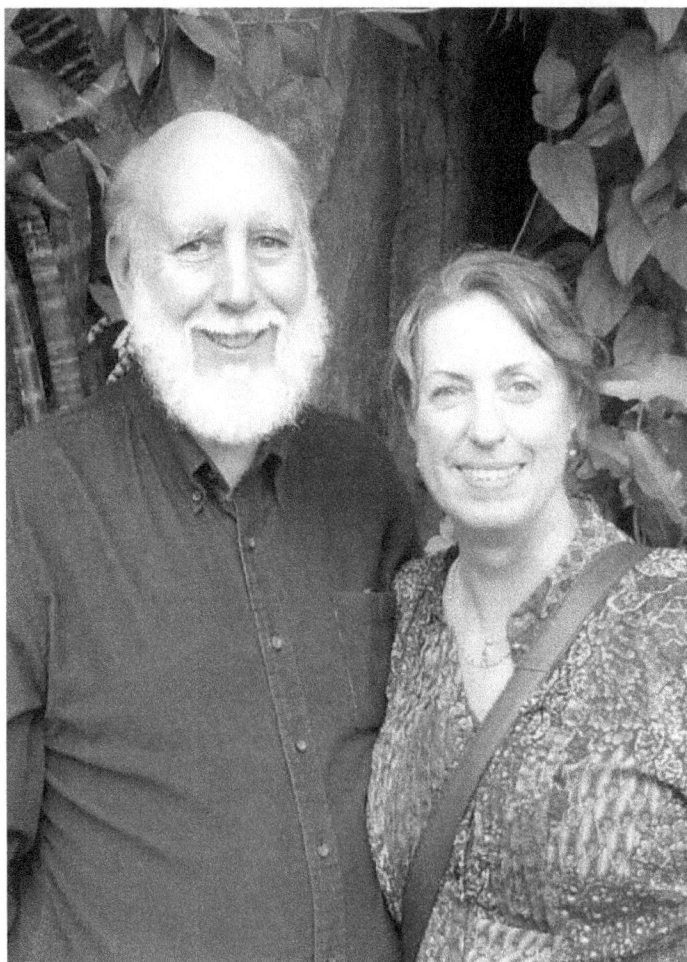

Dr. Raphael d'Angelo and Nancy d'Angelo.

Dr. d'Angelo has spent the biggest part of his medical career in holistic family practice. Most often, he provided natural, complementary and alternative options, saving traditional medical approaches for more rare instances, when they were most needed. Nancy's philosophy fit with his like "hand and glove." A direct quote from Nancy is:

> When you look at the way we are put on this earth, everything the human body needs is coming from the earth. God took care of that. Everything we need is coming from natural resources.

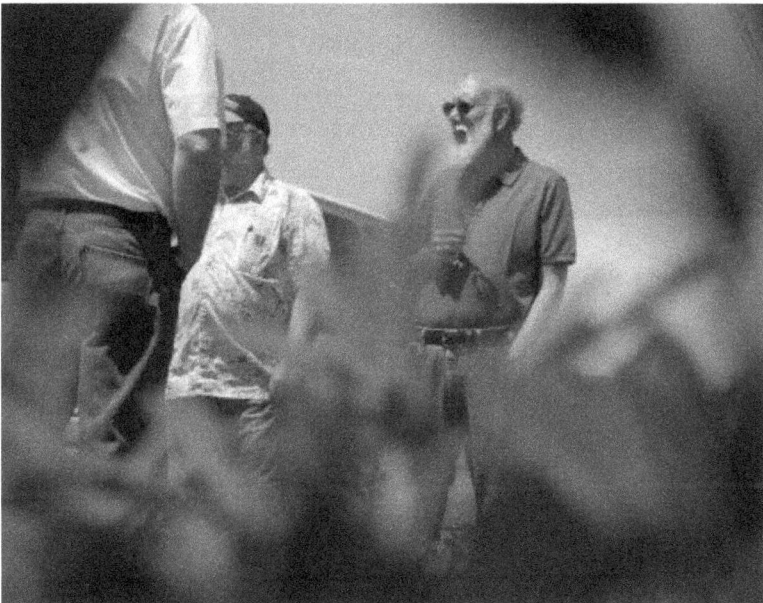

Is it any wonder that these two souls recognized each other? They were yet to discover, through their relationship, that living life in harmony with nature would bring with it surprising transformational qualities to their lives, including an additional residence in Pritchett, Colorado!

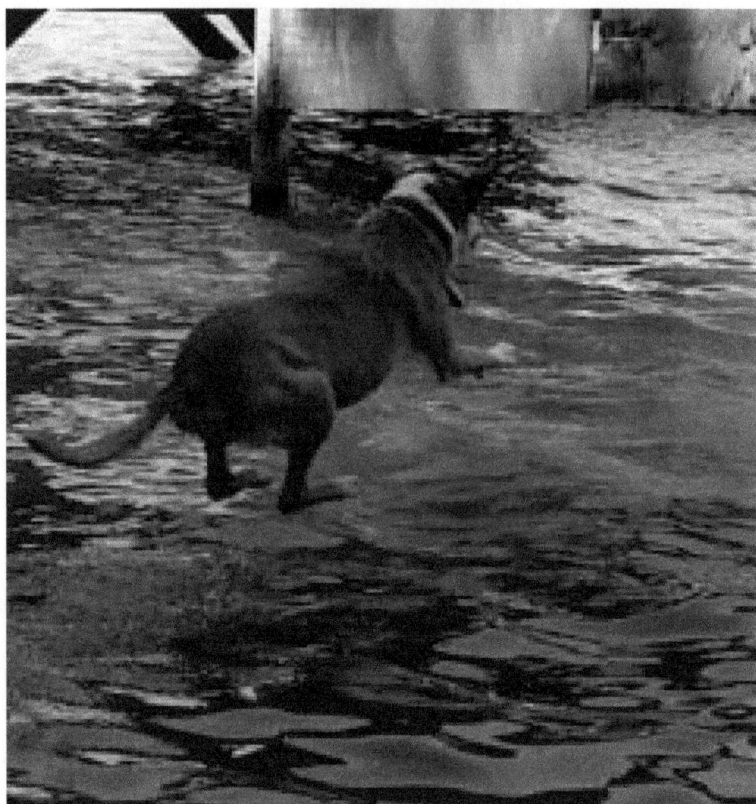

Before her radiation hormesis treatments, Aura's dog Odessa could not jump or move quickly. Today "she's like a new dog."

For their first date, the good doctor invited Nancy out for coffee. She told him, "No thank you. I don't drink coffee. But there is an exhibition at the museum and I would love to go and see it." Nancy says, "From that time forward, we have practically been inseparable."

In the joyful spirit with which Nancy describes marrying the beauty of the fragrance of essential oils with herbology, bringing together the "life blood" of the plant with all of the active chemical constituents, she and Dr. d'Angelo celebrated the joy of their own marriage in 2000.

What Nancy says about her husband:

> He knew from a very early age that he wanted to be a doctor, a healer, someone who helps people. So he acted on it. With his earliest training as a medical technologist in the Air Force, it was sink or swim. He discovered that parasitology work, being in a lab and finding "life" under the microscope lens was something he enjoyed very much. Later, after completing medical school, he combined that early training, keeping his parasitology credentials current, with his family practice which lasted for forty years.

> Keeping him functioning "like a well oiled machine;" taking care of details so he doesn't have to worry; adding my own opinion and bouncing things off of each other to provide the best care for the patient's healing; these are all the things I love to do in support of my husband's work. My husband does think outside the box and I sometimes think further outside the box. I do have a mind of my own and like to use it too!

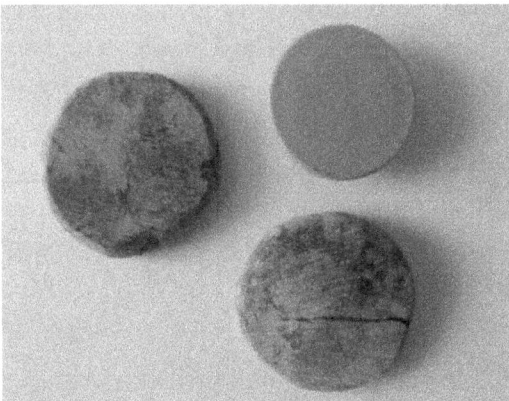

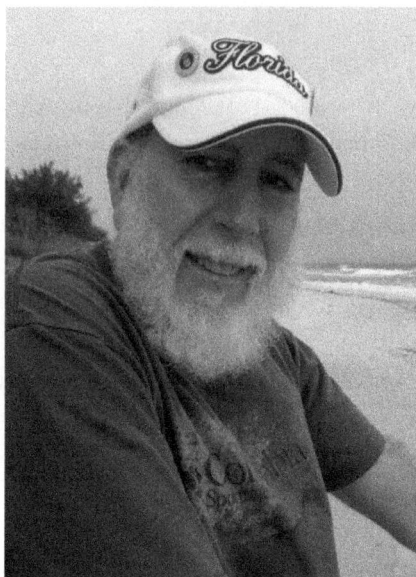

We both agree very strongly, it's important to have several different knowledge bases to pull from and it's just as important to look at an issue from a lot of different angles. This is why working with Jay and Faye, Walt and Kathy, and The Divine Three Protocol is so deeply satisfying to each of us. Each of our parts is critically important to the healing process of our clients. You'll read more about my husband's explanation of the protocol aspects later in this manual. He has an extraordinary way of creating "light bulb moments," making what might otherwise seem difficult to understand, very simple, clear, and poignant at the same time.

What I most want you to know about Raphael d'Angelo is he's a very practical man and very intuitive. And, a more caring treasure I don't think is on this earth.

2

DEFINED ESSENCES, COST, AND REQUIRED ACTIONS TO ACQUIRE EACH PART OF THE DIVINE THREE PROTOCOL

S O WHAT IS THE REAL deal? First of all, it's important to acknowledge the intentions and commitments of these healers. This writer chose the word "musketeers" in Chapter One as a word to describe them, because originally, a musketeer was a "pioneer soldier," committed to fight the toughest battles to bring about the highest good. And, of course, pioneers were the ones who were/are willing to go "out there," where explorations for the truth are not always quick, or simple, or comfortable, in previously traveled territory, or easily understood.

These three couples, each developing their own protocols, have made whatever sacrifices were required, whatever time and energy was needed, and provided whatever support they knew was important for their clients/patients' healing processes, which to date has totaled, all together, over 136 years. There's at least one observation regarding their practices, disciplines, and relationships that is shared by almost everyone who knows them. What every client/patient can count on: "I see you. I hear you. You matter."

DESCRIPTION OF THE DIVINE THREE PROTOCOL
Radiation hormesis, defined by the leading scientists of the 1940s, and 1950s:

> Low doses of natural radiation stimulate rather than destroy. As it travels through the body, low level natural radiation stresses cells and DNA to promote the duplication and repair of healthy cells. No one has ever proven that low doses of natural radiation are harmful. In fact, quite the opposite was discovered as far back as the 1800s, as is clear from the studies of such eminent scientists as Dr. Charles Sanders and T. D. Luckey.

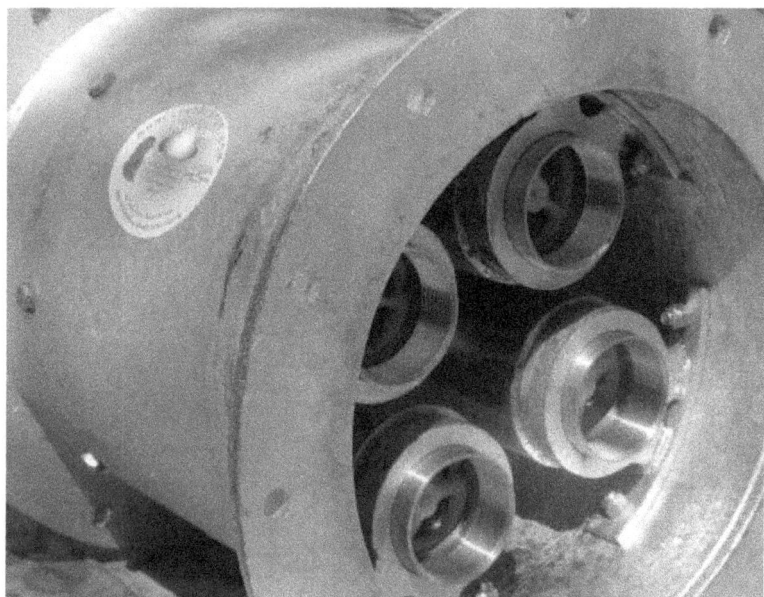

Dr. Sanders' research showed that low dose natural radiation activates a system of transient protective processes that includes antioxidants, high efficiency DNA repair, immunosurveillance—a monitoring process of the immune system which detects and destroys neoplastic cells (an abnormal mass of tissue resulting from an abnormal proliferation of cells) and apoptosis (the process of programmed cell death that may occur in multicellular organisms). The results have been shown to enhance biological responses for immune systems, enzymatic repair, physiological functions, and the removal of cellular damage, including prevention and removal of cancers and other diseases.

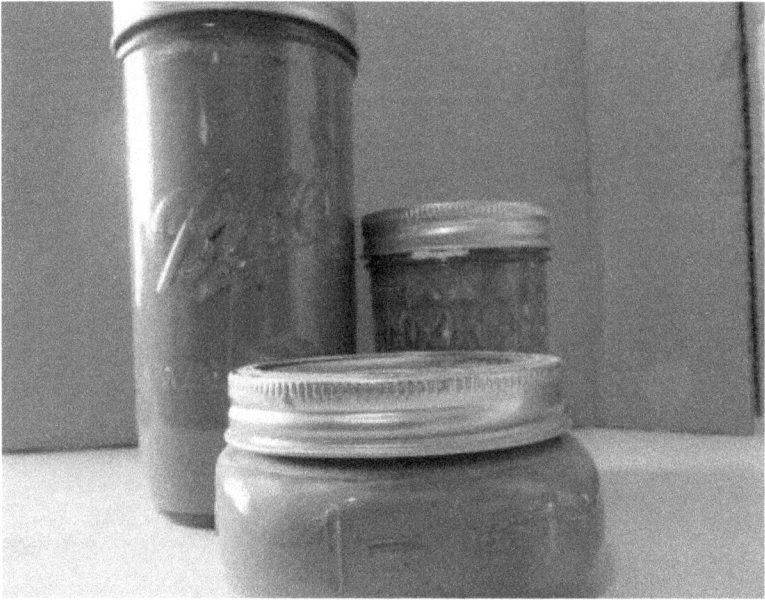

RADIATION HORMESIS FREQUENCIES AS DEFINED BY JAY GUTIERREZ, FOUNDER, CHIEF MEDICINE MAN, & RESEARCHER OF NIGHT HAWK MINERALS

Everything is energy. Energy emits frequencies: a repeating pattern which identifies the energy. Natural radiation, found in nature, come from alpha, beta, and gamma radiation. The radiation waves are made up of many different elements having different numbers of neutrons. All of these different possible versions of each element are called isotopes. The natural radiation energies of all these different isotopes emits frequencies which then imprint themselves on whatever they contact.

Low levels of natural radiation have been proven to have a life-giving, nourishing and healing capacity. "They can be found everywhere in nature and I have discovered them in some particular rocks. When one such rock is dropped in water, the frequencies emitted from the radiation in the rock imprint themselves on water molecules they touch." The imprinted molecules spread to imprint other water molecules so that the entire body of water becomes totally restructured with life-giving frequencies.

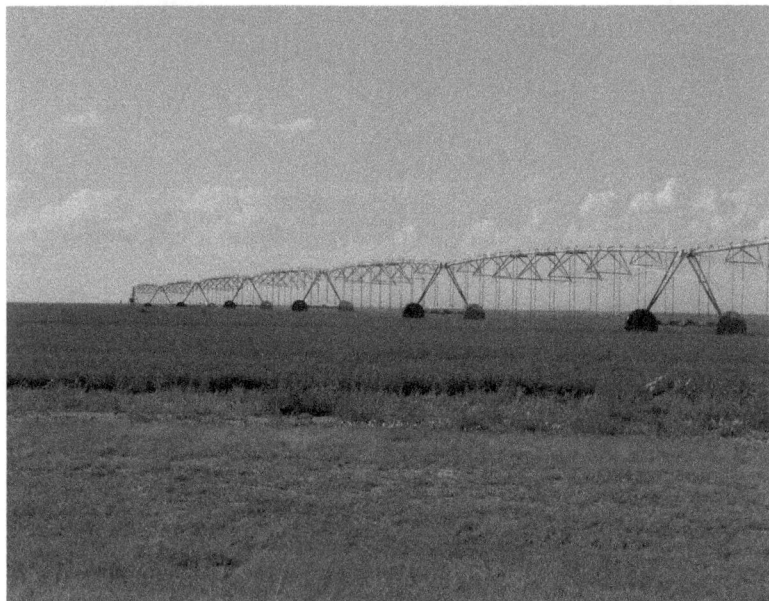

Radiation hormesis frequencies were, as of the summer of 2012, helping a number of beekeepers in Virginia to bring their hives back from the disaster of colony collapse disorder. Two years later, in 2014, honey bees continue to disappear across the country at an alarming rate, putting $15 billion worth of fruits, nuts, and vegetables at risk, according to the USDA. Beekeepers have been reporting this growing disaster since 2006.

Why are the bees vanishing? Scientists studying the disorder believe a combination of factors could be the cause, including pesticide exposure, invasive parasitic mites, an inadequate food supply and a new virus that targets bees' immune systems. Whatever the cause, this group of beekeepers in Virginia now provides water for their bees to drink that is being continually imprinted with radiation hormesis frequencies. The colony collapse disorder has vanished. The bees are finding their way back to the hive. If you know a beekeeper who needs help, have them call Jay at Night Hawk Minerals.

One last example from Jay:

> We have created a sauna/hot stones frequencies
> room at the Mineral Palace. The walls of this room
> are covered with small slices of hot [low
> radioactive] stones. When you sit in a chair in this
> room and turn on the steam diffuser, the steam gets

imprinted with the radiation hormesis frequencies emitted from the hot stones. As you breathe the imprinted molecules of air, and as your skin absorbs the imprinted frequencies, your lungs and your body become infused with the healing energy of radiation hormesis frequencies. Your body can begin to heal.

WATER DIVINE: THE 5 STEP SYSTEM TO OPTIMIZE YOUR HEALTH — BEYOND BEING PHYSICALLY FIT, FOLLOW THESE STEPS TO BECOME HEALTHY

Walt and Kathy Merriman have "designed" truly divine pure water by adding water soluble, naturally ionized, angstrom sized minerals. Minerals and vitamins are two of the most important nutrients known to man. They have a chain like dependency. One mineral depends on another mineral, which depends on a vitamin and so on. We call this synergy. The wellness of your body is only as strong as the weakest link in the chain.

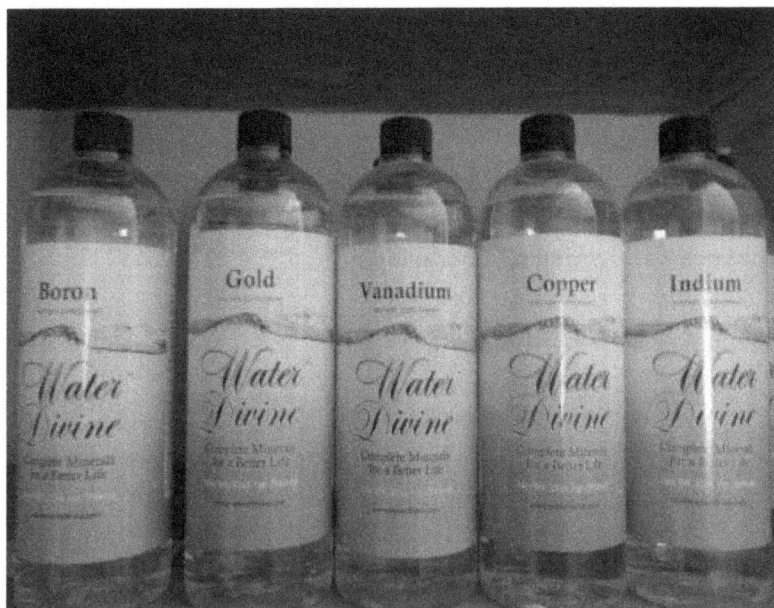

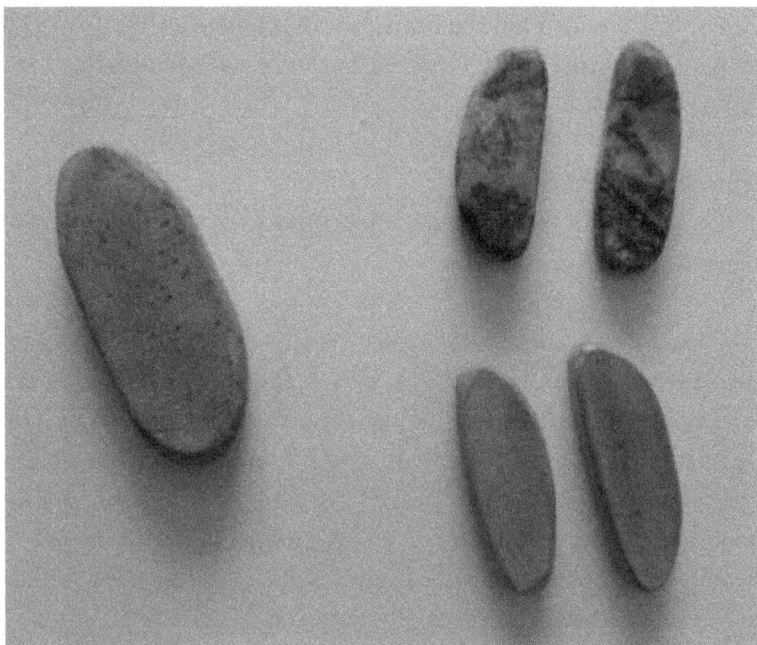

STEP 1: COMPLETE BODY FOUNDATION KIT
This liquid nutrition system combines 70-plus essential and trace minerals, as well as Vitamins A, B, C, D, and E, along with the amino acids, into the Water Divine flagship product. Understand, if a person is deficient in just one mineral or vitamin it could compromise the body's ability to heal itself.

STEP 2: THE COMPLETE CLEANSE KIT
You must remove the toxins that have weakened your immune system and that created an environment which allows diseases to live and grow. Some of the cleanses it includes are a Colon, Liver and Gall Bladder Cleanse, Toxic Sludge, Arterial and Heart Valve, Heavy Metal, and even a Fat Cell Cleanse for those concerned about their Blood Sugar Wellness. The Divine Three Protocol program focuses on the Colon, Liver and Gall Bladder Cleanses. Also, there are over 8,000 different species of parasites that are

known to have invaded the human body. Consider that parasites eat us, then expel their waste in us. We call this waste, toxic sludge.

STEP 3: EXERCISE
As you complete Steps one and two, you will have the necessary energy to feel like exercising.

Exercise for mind, body and spirit, is critical for physical, mental, and spiritual development and well being. In the martial arts training of this writer, learning to flow physically, mentally, and spiritually teaches self-discipline, control, and it improves health. Exercise develops strength, power, balance, coordination, agility, flexibility, and endurance. As a discipline, a commitment to exercise develops qualities of patience, perseverance, and humility. More information in the area of exercise is in Section 8.

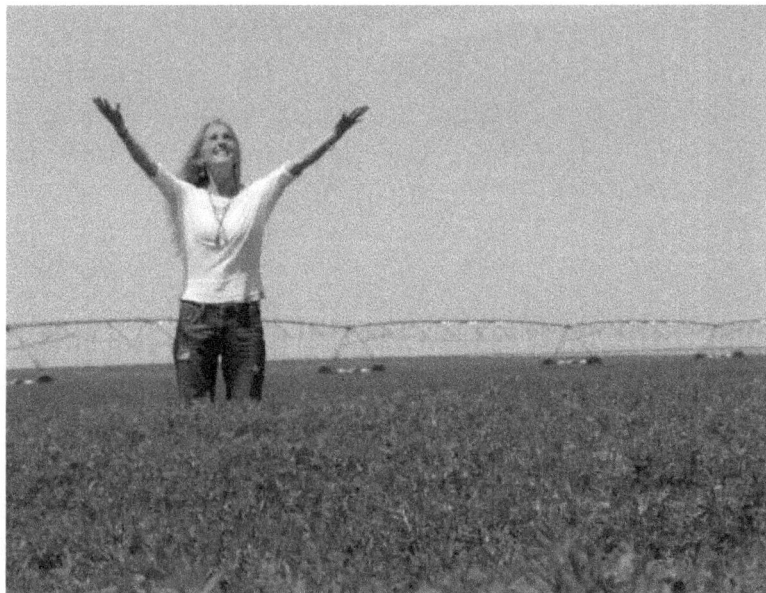

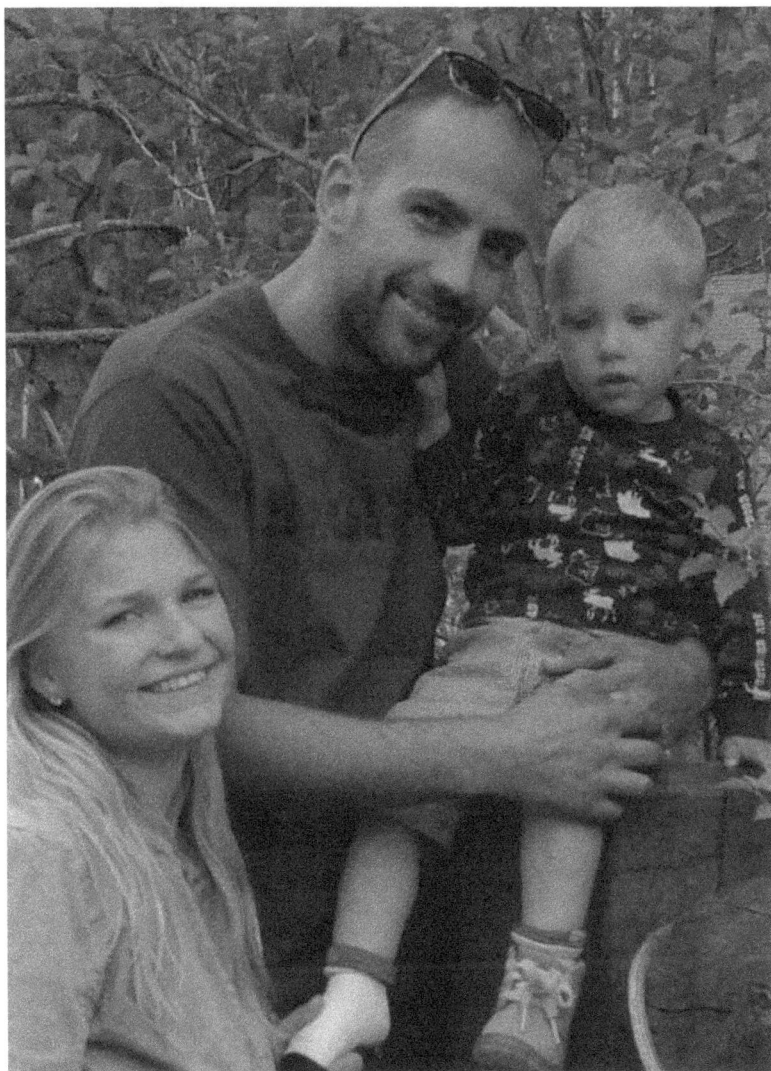

The Cox family, owners of Levi's Bed and Breakfast: Vanessa, Daniel, and Emmett.

STEP 4: MONITOR PH

Few diseases can live or survive when the body's pH level is where it needs to be! Therefore, when you learn how to maintain a pH level of 7.4 without manipulation of your body, it's very difficult to get sick. And, when you do maintain the pH, the body will be positioned to quickly heal itself. One of the keys to living in a state of "Wellness" is to monitor your pH level. Drugstores carry litmus paper to test saliva and urine. It's simple to find all natural alkaline diet information in the library and/or the internet.

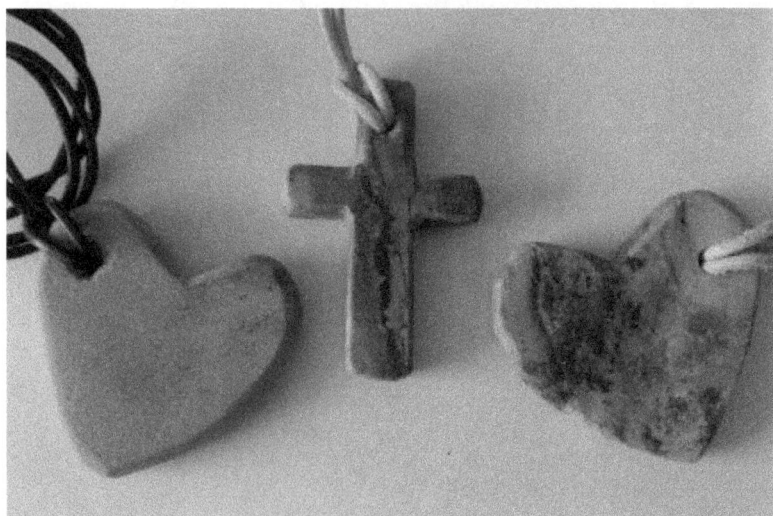

STEP 5: TARGET SPECIFIC AREAS THAT NEED HEALING
When the body has the right minerals, the body has a better chance of healing itself. Therefore, once you learn what mineral(s) your body is deficient in, and you get the right mineral(s), the body will heal itself! Targeting an organ or gland with extra nutrition is the key to increase healing.

Walt's knowledge and information on each mineral will help you understand and apply this process easily. Water Divine's contact information is on the Contact Information page of this manual.

PARAWELLNESS RESEARCH: THE IDENTIFICATION AND ELIMINATION OF PARASITES
Dr. d'Angelo's earliest medical training in the Air force led him to Vietnam for a year. As a Medical Technologist working in

Microbiology and Parasitology, he saw under the microscope lens what was devastating our GIs and was fascinated with the ways he could diagnose those organisms. When Jay and Dr. d'Angelo met in 2006, Jay did not know that Dr. d'Angelo had kept his Parasitology credentials current during his entire 40 year medical family practice.

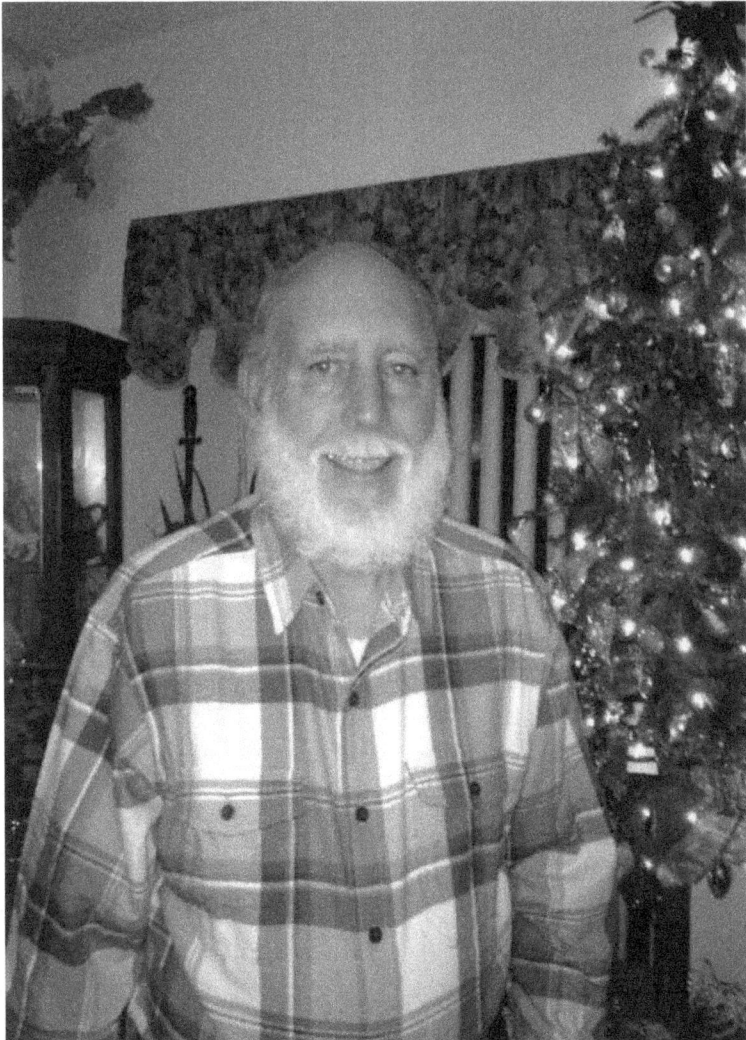

Dr. d'Angelo.

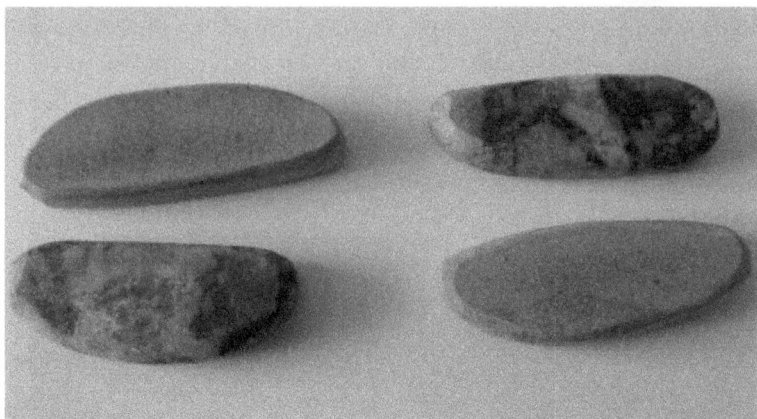

It seemed like divine intervention as Jay realized in 2010 that the expense of sending parasite test samples to Nigeria was no longer feasible. He needed to find the support "close to home." As Dr. d'Angelo was closing his family practice, it came as a wonderful surprise when Jay learned that he was a licensed Parasitologist and his credentials were current. So in May of 2011, Dr. d'Angelo accepted Jay's offer to also be the Night Hawk Minerals Parasitologist, as well as Medical Director.

It's a 4-step process to experience the ParaWellness program:

1. When you request a parasite test kit from Dr. d'Angelo, it is shipped to you.
2. You collect stool and urine samples according to the directions in the test kit and return the kit to Dr. d'Angelo.
3. A phone appointment is set up for Dr. d'Angelo to discuss the results of the tests, answer questions, and provide the remedies as needed.
4. Because the remedies target parasite eggs and larvae, as well as the full grown worms, yeast, and protozoans, you begin a three month cycle for taking remedies specific to what parasites were found. Depending on the extent of

infestation of particular parasites, you will be guided by Dr. d'Angelo who will determine if additional cycles of parasite elimination are required.

Within The Divine Three Protocol, the parasite program frees up the immune system from having to deal with the very difficult parasite load, so that it can accomplish its task of taking care of other conditions, such as a cancer. If the immune system is busy treating parasites, it is not taking as much time and function to eliminate the cancer. So the parasite program fits in to help release the immune system to go and do its job. It also stops tissue destruction and the resulting toxic sludge, which is caused by parasite activity.

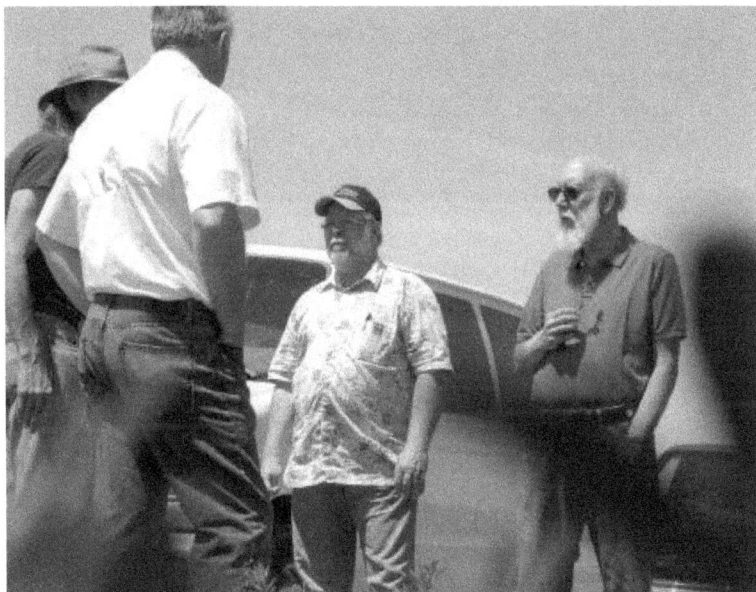

Jay far left, Dr. d'Angelo far right.

Dr. d'Angelo helps us see the bigger picture. When you bring in an energy like radiation hormesis frequencies, and you have the right mineral load, this means the minerals act like liquid wires which set up the paths to the cells. The radiation hormesis frequencies excite and imprint on the minerals. The minerals then carry the action of the frequencies to the cells of the body and that is extremely important for the healing process to take place.

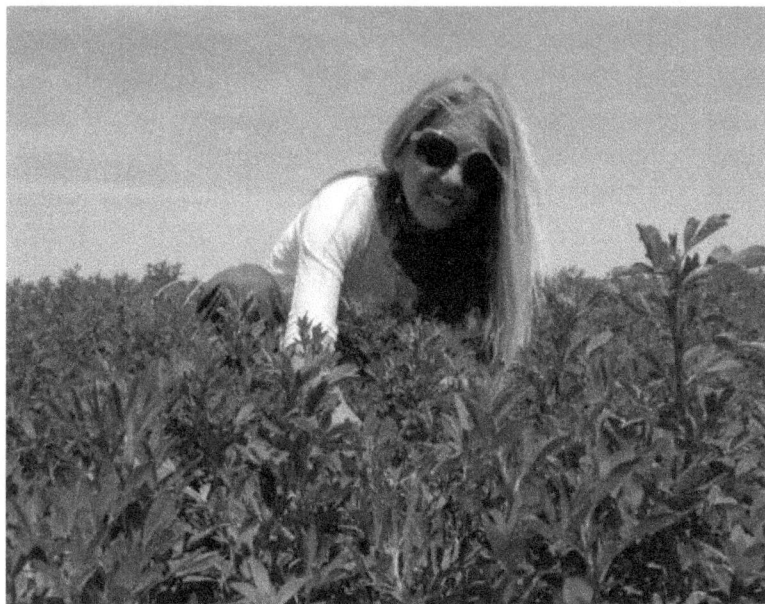

If you do not have the right mineral balance, you can have all the remedies you want to take care of all the parasites, but the person does not function well. The different organs are not optimally working, so it's very important to have all three aspects: 1) free up the immune system, 2) have the energy frequencies coming in through the stones being carried on the mineral pathway of liquid wires, which 3) take the healing energy to the cells. Every aspect comes from the earth's natural resources. That's divine healing. That's The Divine Three Protocol.

COSTS AND ACTIONS TO TAKE TO ACQUIRE THE DIVINE THREE PROTOCOL
Being cost effective without jeopardizing quality is very important to us. Most people calling us for help have been hit hard by the

economy, and also, in many cases, have been financially drained from mainstream medical bills, or have exhausted their funds purchasing a myriad of natural wellness products that ultimately, did not offer much promise.

Jay speaks adamantly:

> Don't get me wrong, there are many good natural products out there, but without guidance and because other pieces of the puzzle are so often missing, they are usually not fully addressing the problem.

The Divine Three Protocol is designed so that between the three different support groups—stones, minerals, and parasite testing and elimination—the full protocol is about $1,500. If the health issue is at a life-threatening critical stage, and finances are already a challenge, The Divine Three Protocol can be broken up into stages, making it affordable.

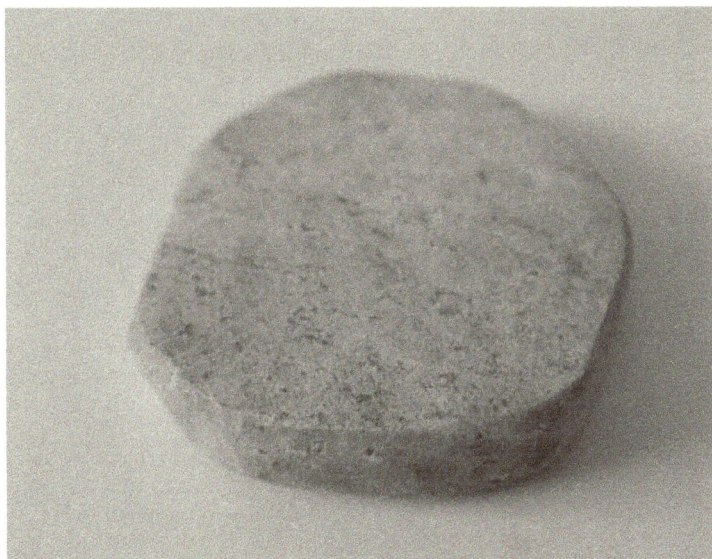

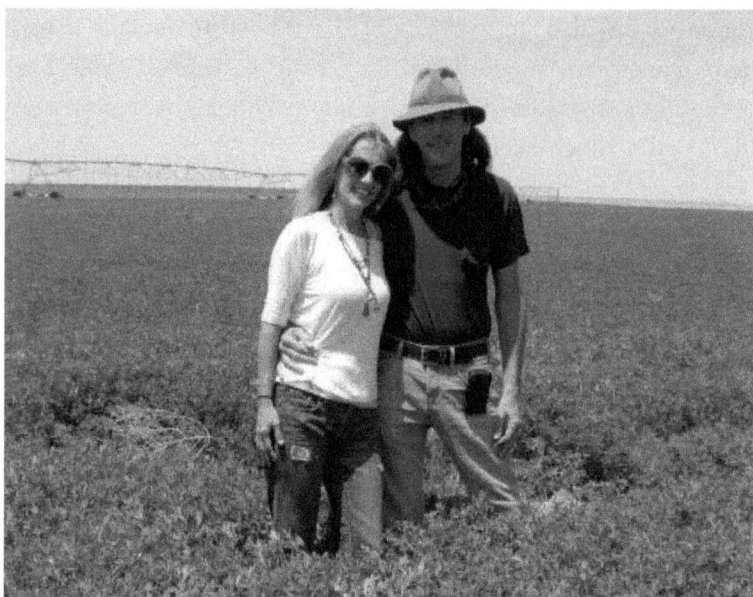

The action to take: Contact Night Hawk Minerals. The contact information for all three protocol groups is on the Contact Information page. Following Jay's instructions:

> Begin working with your Night Hawk Minerals Wellness Instructor so that we can keep things in sequence for you. Pay attention to your body's responses, and direct other issues that may arise to the right support group within our circle. Over time, we are certain that prices will change, but not in a way that would keep The Divine Three Protocol out of the hands of those who need it. If you need help, please do not hesitate to contact us! God Bless. Jay Gutierrez, Night Hawk Minerals/Founder

3

THE STEPS TO HEALING USING THE DIVINE THREE PROTOCOL

IT'S HELPFUL TO REMEMBER THE Divine Three Protocol can be used at any time, by anyone without harmful effects. In addition to targeting degenerative diseases, it is actually an excellent health and wellness booster to go through at least once a year, with the exception of the Foundation Kit minerals, and the Night Hawk Minerals Kit stones and Mudpack, which are meant to be a part of your daily life for health maintenance.

Getting started combines the processes of using radiation hormesis frequencies and mineralization of the body with Water Divine. This combination is important because of the synchronicity of healing energies which begin to restructure the abilities of cells to reach a state of "homeostasis." Because the frequencies and mineralization are working interactively in the body, this helps you achieve a greater balanced state towards whatever parts of the body most need healing.

STEP 1
Receive your Radiation Hormesis Kit, and Hot Stone. The instructions and brochure in the kit give you details about using the

Pendant Stone, Water Stone, Green Stone and Mudpack. After in-depth consultation, the level of millirems (mRm) of radiation in the hot stone—level one, two, or three—will be designated by your personal Night Hawk Minerals Wellness Instructor. Begin using the stones as directed. Contact information for Wellness Instructors is on the Contact Information page.

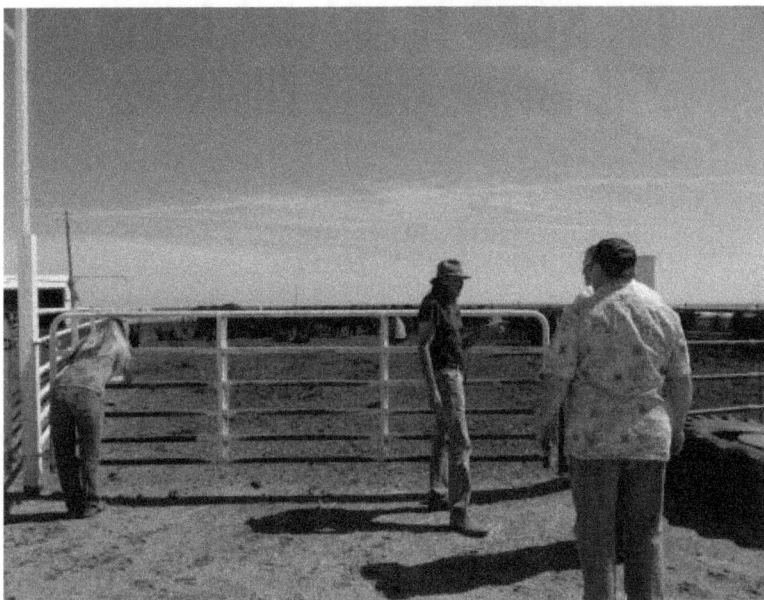

After three days of using the stones, call your Wellness Instructor and report what you are experiencing. Check in with questions and feedback, numerous times, with your Wellness Instructor. This initiative, on your part, is critically important to your success in the program. The Night Hawk Minerals Medical Director, Dr. Raphael d'Angelo, along with Jay Gutierrez, will provide supervision and consultation with your Wellness Instructor for individuals who have been diagnosed with advanced stages of a myriad of degenerative diseases.

STEP 2

As you begin using the radiation hormesis stones, at the same time, also begin using the Water Divine Complete Foundation Kit. This liquid nutrition system is the result of many years of research and experience applying these food supplements to the diets of average people. You will be taking a special blend of thirteen of the body's most needed essential trace minerals, as well as many more adding up to a total of 70-plus minerals, and a powerful organic liquid multivitamin, consisting of A, B, C, D and E, plus essential amino acids and more.

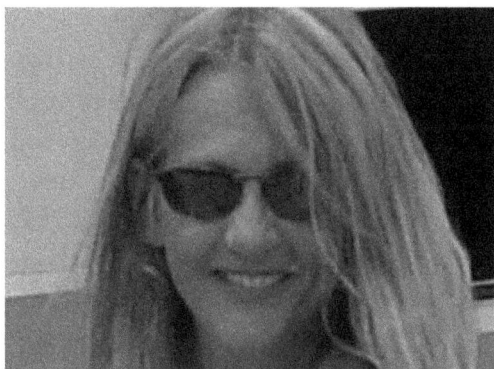

You will follow the directions on each of the 3 bottles: Adults take 1 tablespoon per day, children take ½ tablespoon (1 teaspoon) per day. Walt recommends infants or toddlers take 1 drop for each one pound of body weight from each of the 3 bottles: Essentials, Mag-Cal, and Potas-Zin.

At the same time you are taking the Complete Body Foundation Kit minerals as directed with instructions inside the box, you will need to drink water: ½ of your body weight in ounces per day, every day. Example: A person who weighs 120 pounds would drink 60 ounces of water each day. Your juices, coffee, teas, and beer do not count as your water intake. The radiation hormesis Water Stone should be allowed to charge the water you drink for at least eight hours before you begin drinking the stone water. The radiation hormesis stone water and reverse osmosis filtered water are the types of water you should be drinking.

STEP 3
As close to the first day, or before the first day, you begin your Divine Three Protocol using the Radiation Hormesis Kit stones and Mudpack, and taking the liquid mineral and vitamin nutrients of the Water Divine Complete Body Foundation Kit, you will order your Parawellness Research Program parasite test kit.

As soon as possible, send in your stool and urine samples to Dr. d'Angelo in Aurora, Colorado. Based on multiple microscopic examinations of your samples, within 7 to 14 days of receiving your test samples, you will receive a booklet of results information with which to set up a phone consultation with Dr. d'Angelo. During the consultation, Dr. d'Angelo will explain the results, answer your questions, and make recommendations for remedies. At your request, the recommended remedies will be sent to you by UPS.

STEP 4
After a minimum of 10 days of using the radiation hormesis stones kit and taking the Water Divine liquid nutrients, you will begin the first two cleanses using the Water Divine Body Cleanse Kit.

The first cleanse targets the liver and colon. The second cleanse targets the gall bladder. The second cleanse should immediately follow the first and both cleanses will be completed within a total of two days. There are alternative instructions, on page 28, for anyone who is too weak to complete the cleanse so quickly. While Dr. d'Angelo's parasite remedies target yeast, parasites and protozoans, these cleanses are intended to clear the bile ducts and lymph system, and allow the body to eliminate toxins and food waste. If these cleanses

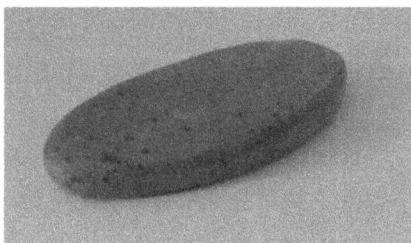

are not attended to, as the parasites are killed off, with the 3rd protocol—Dr. d'Angelo's parasite remedies—the sludge can build up in the body, creating more toxins, thus more problems.

CLEANSE 1: LIVER/COLON CLEANSE

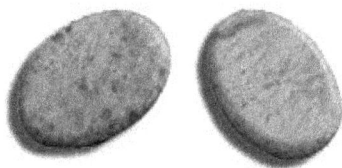

Note about the elderly and very weak: These individuals will follow different instructions and a 19 day schedule which is outlined in the next few pages.

Using the complete body foundation minerals for at least ten days prior to this cleanse will do at least two things:

a. Help the body stay hydrated.
b. Help avoid possible leg cramping from having magnesium and electrolyte deficiencies.

• This cleanse is for adults only.
• This is a 24-hour rapid cleanse of the colon and liver.
• It's very effective, yet may be too harsh for some individual's systems, especially the elderly and very weak.
• If completed, you may see large volumes of light green stones passed, ranging from bb size to small marble size.
• Continue to use the foundation minerals and vitamins each day of the cleanse to help with hydration.

What you will need (this is enough for 2 people):

1. Cleanse-O Plus Powder (in the Cleanse Kit).
2. 7 oz. bottle of olive oil, extra virgin cold pressed.
3. ½ gallon pink or red grapefruit juice (preferable to use unsweetened, not from concentrate).
4. An open schedule—no plans—the evening of day 1 and the

morning of day 2.

5. A lubricant is recommended, such as Vaseline, between bathroom breaks to prevent chaffing.

6. Drink lots of water to stay hydrated, reverse osmosis filtered water if possible, and radiation hormesis stone water, which has been charged for 8 hours, or more, before drinking.

7. Continue to use the Complete Body Foundation Kit each day of the cleanse to help with hydration.

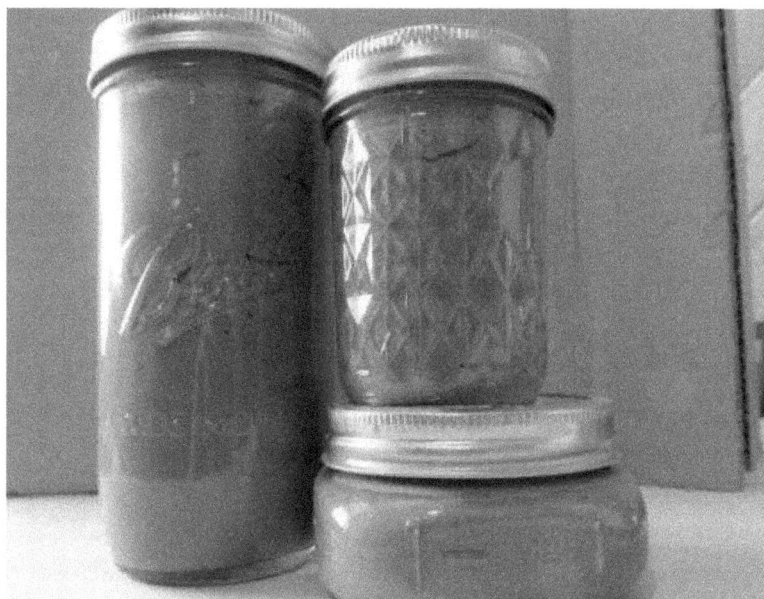

INSTRUCTIONS TO COMPLETE THE CLEANSE
Day 1

1. If possible, begin the cleanse with a day of fasting. It is okay to take the Complete Body Foundation Kit minerals and vitamins on the days of the fast. On the first day, if you must eat, only eat a light breakfast.

2. For a body weight of 150 pounds or less, mix 1 level tablespoon of Cleanse-O Plus into 4 oz. of water and 4 oz. of grapefruit juice. For a body weight over 150 pounds, mix 2 level tablespoons of Cleanse-O Plus into 4 oz. of water and 4 oz. of grapefruit juice.

3. At 4 PM, on the day of the fast, drink the above appropriate mixture of Cleanse-O Plus/water/grapefruit juice. Drink it all.

4. At 6 PM on the same fasting day, place 1 teaspoon of Cleanse-O Plus in the mixture of 4 oz. of water and 4 oz. of grapefruit juice. Drink it all.

5. At 10:00 PM mix 4 oz. of cold pressed olive oil with 4 oz. of pink or red grapefruit juice. Stir very fast and drink with a straw. Go to bed immediately for your night's sleep.

Day 2
6. At 8:00 AM drink another 8 oz. mixture of water, grapefruit

juice, and 1 teaspoon of Cleanse-O Plus.

7. At 10:00 AM start drinking the apple juice (one gallon of pure apple juice—no sugar added). Throughout the day, consume as much of the gallon of apple juice as you can before bedtime.

INSTRUCTIONS FOR THE ELDERLY AND VERY WEAK INDIVIDUALS
This more gentle cleanse will last for 19 days.

What you will need:
a. Unsweetened juices: lemon, lime, grapefruit, cranberry.
b. Tea bags: milk thistle, ginger, red clover, dandelion.
c. Cleanse-O Plus from the cleanse kit.
d. Extra virgin, cold pressed olive oil.

1. Every night, before bed for 5 days: take 1 oz. of olive oil mixed with 3 oz. of unsweetened juice. Rotate the juices as listed above,

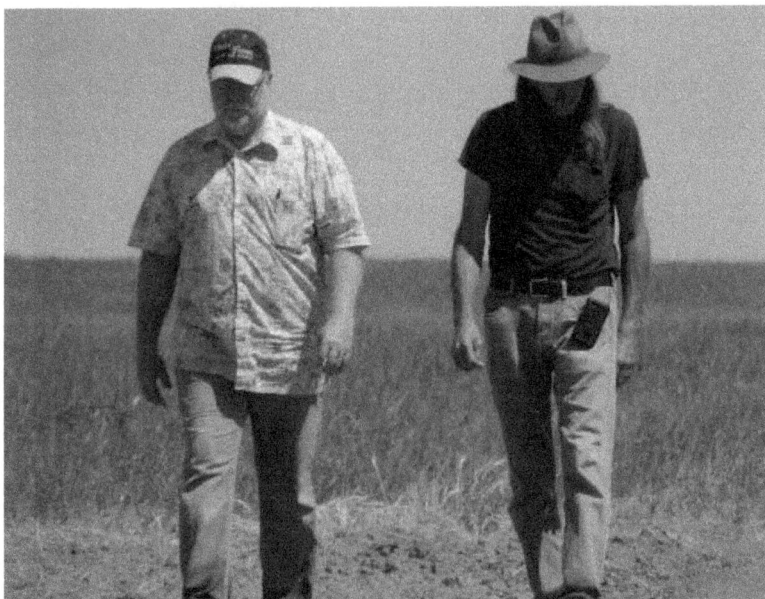

in the order they are listed.

2. If the bowels do not loosen by the second day, drink a mixture of 1 heaping teaspoon of Cleanse-O Plus with unsweetened juice after a light breakfast.
3. For the next two weeks, only every other day, drink the same juice/olive oil mixture, rotating the juices.

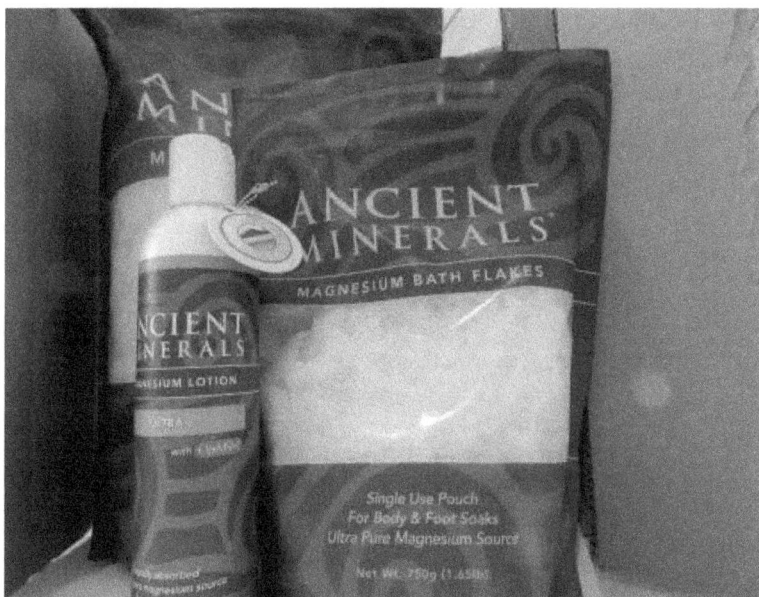

4. During these same two weeks, on the same days (every other day) that you are drinking the juice/olive oil mixture, also drink 2 cups of warm tea—one in the early morning and one in the late evening before bed.

The tea should be 4 cups of water with 4 tea bags—one tea bag of each listed above. No microwave is to be used in making the tea.

STEP 5: CLEANSE 2: GALL BLADDER CLEANSE
Notes:
• This is also a 24-hour cleanse and is more effective immediately
    after the liver cleanse because the bowel is already empty.
• This cleanse is helpful even if the gall bladder has been removed.
• Hunger will not be a problem.

What you will need:
a. 1 gal. of pure apple juice (no sugar added).
b. 17 oz. bottle of extra virgin, cold pressed olive oil—use what's
    left from the liver cleanse.
c. Lemon juice - fresh or real lemon concentrate.

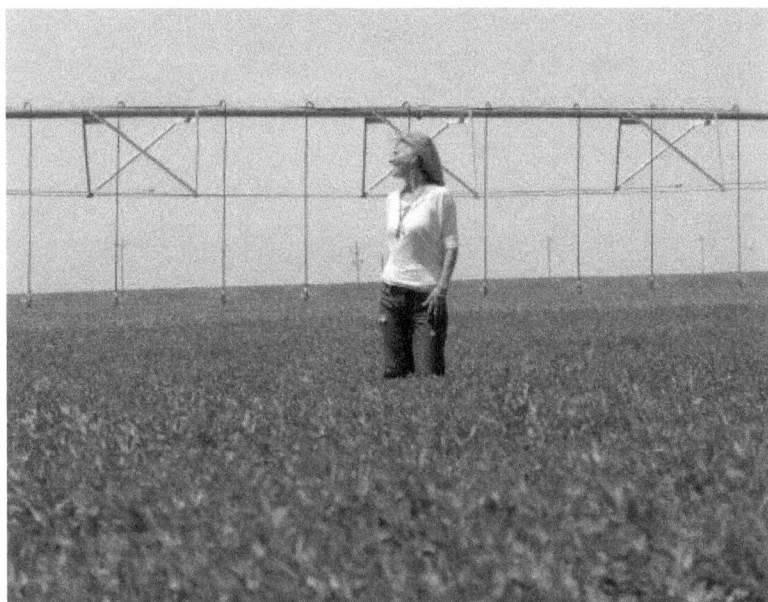

Note: Special instructions if you have diabetes: Substitute 2
medium-sized apples and 32 oz. of apple juice mixed with 3 quarts
of water. Drink slowly and keep track of your sugar levels.

Instructions to complete the cleanse:

Day 1:

1. It's best to begin this cleanse on the second day of the liver/colon cleanse. Start drinking pure apple juice early in the day, even as you are still taking the Cleanse-O Plus from the liver cleanse. Eat no food. Consume as much of the gallon of apple juice as you can before bedtime.

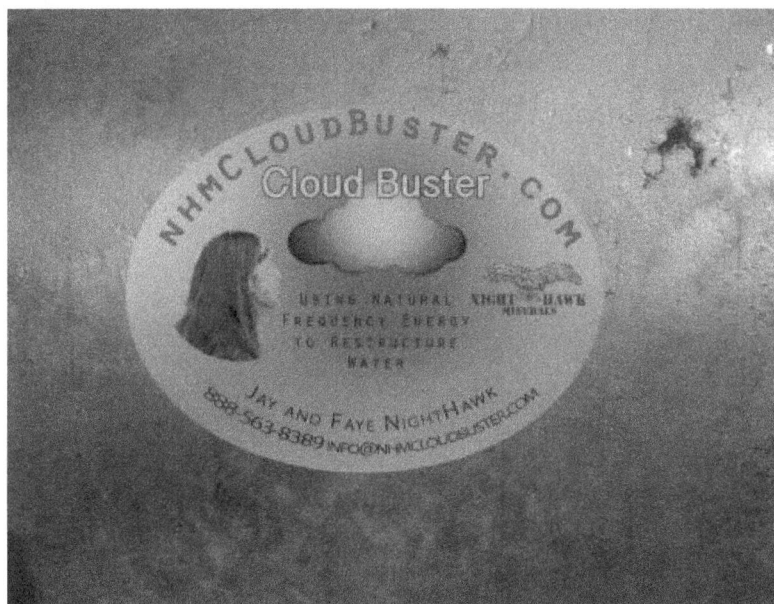

2. At bedtime, drink a mixture of 4 oz. olive oil with 4 oz. lemon juice. This works best if you stir very fast and drink with a straw.

Day 2:

3. Upon arising, you will likely pass completely different colored stones that will be a darker green color. You may begin eating when you feel like it.

STEP 6

Now you're ready to begin the three month cycle of Dr. d'Angelo's parasite remedies. While you are continuing to use the RH Kit stones and take the Water Divine nutrients, you will begin the three month cycle of Dr. d'Angelo's parasite specific remedies targeting yeast, particular parasites and protozoans.

The directions for taking the parasite remedies are included in your report booklet sent to you with the results of testing. Depending on the extent of infestation of particular parasites, you will be guided by Dr. d'Angelo who will determine if additional cycles of parasite elimination are required.

STEP 7

At the completion of the liver, colon, and gall bladder cleanses, your body is now better prepared for the eliminations to occur as you proceed with the 3 month cycle of parasite remedies specifically targeting your particular parasites. It is highly recommended for you to continue using the radiation hormesis kit stones and continue to take the Water Divine Complete Body Foundation Kit minerals and vitamins to increase the experiences of vitality, energy and overall well being.

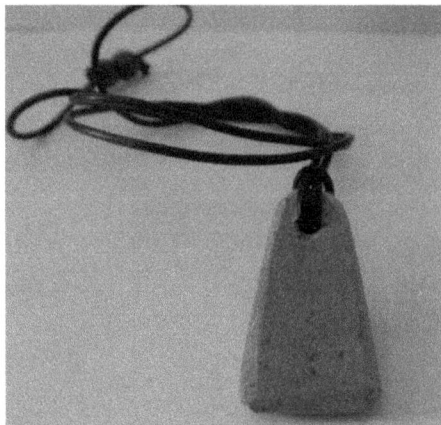

4

FREQUENTLY ASKED QUESTIONS AND ANSWERS ABOUT THE DIVINE THREE PROTOCOL

YOU MAY HAVE QUESTIONS THAT have not been covered thus far. In order to reach the practitioners of The Divine Three Protocol, their individual contact information, along with the contact information of each Wellness Instructor, is on the Contact Information page of this manual. They will appreciate hearing from you by email, as well as by phone. On emails, please add your phone number so follow up contact can include phone conversations as needed.

The individual Websites representing each part of The Divine Three Protocol also present Frequently Asked Questions and Answers on their websites. The Website addresses are also on the Contact Information page.

So many times, Night Hawk Minerals Wellness Instructors are talking with clients who are "at the end of their rope." If you are questioning whether to "tie a knot and hang on" or let go, make sure you talk with a Wellness Instructor before you decide. Your

Wellness Instructor will work with you, based on what you are feeling, and give you encouragement to support your will to live. Our Medical Director, Dr. d'Angelo has learned in over thirty-five years of practice, a person's will to live makes the greatest difference in what direction their life goes.

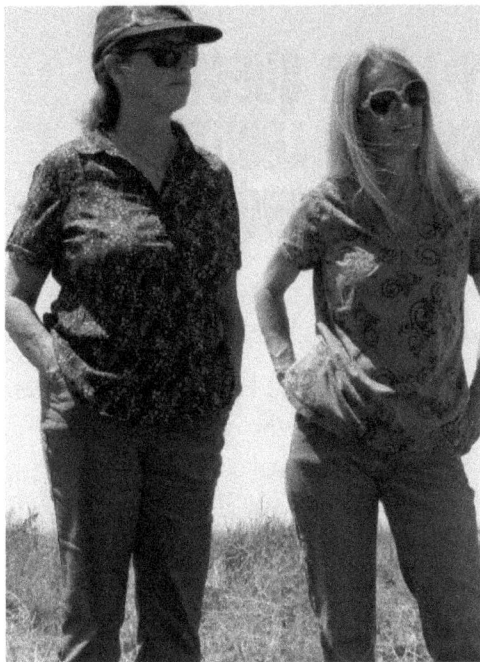

Nancy d'Angelo and Faye Gutierrez.

Q: If your question is: What do I do because I am losing my will to live?

A: Pick up the phone and call someone you know will help you. Our medical staff and Wellness Instructors at Night Hawk Minerals are here to guide you in making decisions that will focus on healing your body, mind, and spirit. Please feel free to call us. Contact information is in Section 9.

Q: Will the Night Hawk Minerals radiation hurt me?

A: Here at Night Hawk Minerals we have been working with low dose naturally radiated ore for years. We have also been backed by the research completed by scientists, a nuclear physicist, and doctors who are our friends, and who are recognized as the world's experts. They even come visit us! Over this time, we have always tried to align their theories on radiation hormesis with the miracles we have witnessed. It was difficult. Now, we have seen with our own eyes, and it is our position that it is the *frequencies* that are accomplishing these feats of healing, among many other things.

Natural radiation is different than the radiation you would receive in a hospital, which is radiation that has been altered. We believe that natural radiation which has been artificially altered becomes an untruth. We have *never* had anyone that was in any way traumatized when using these frequencies over the years. Ourselves, we don't get sick very often.

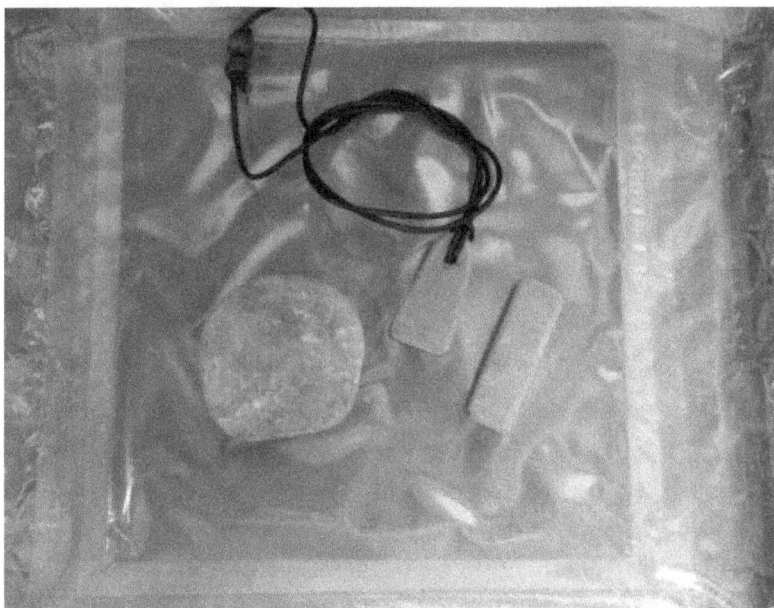

Q: Will the Night Hawk Minerals radiation help with *my* condition?
A: From what *we* have observed, progress has been made with every degenerative disease we have worked with. We have validated that these frequencies *always* make the *right move*! The main thing is to stay consistent with your protocol, and let your Wellness Instructor know of any body responses you experience. We will guide you along this process.

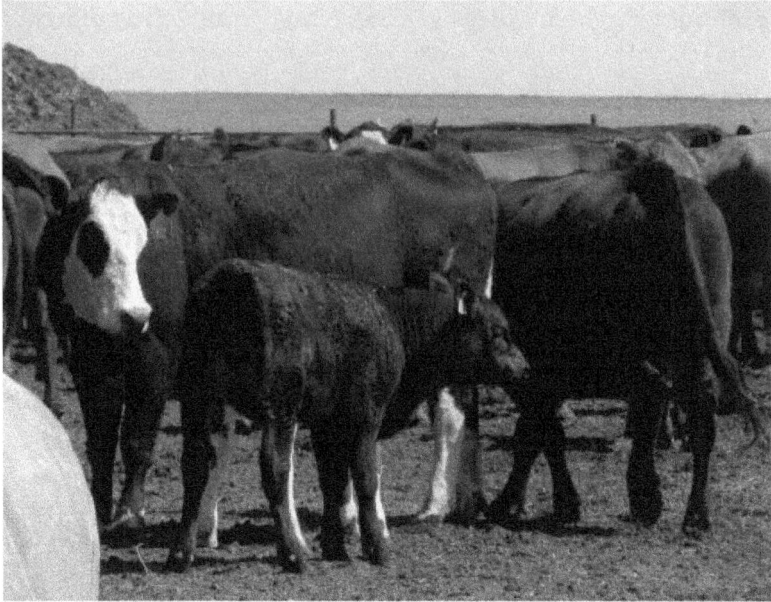

Radiation hormesis treated water helped these cows regain their health.

Q: Can I talk to someone who has gone through this before and used The Divine Three Protocol?

A: Because of how we have to conduct business, we do not give out information on or from our other clients, unless it is a special case, and we have their permission. We have done this in the past, but do not make it a habit. As far as all that we have *seen*, our methods and therapeutic agents, inclusive of The Divine Three Protocol, seem to be working with the best success rate of any other program we know about.

Q: How soon will The Divine Three Protocol start working?

A: Even though every individual is different, most people start getting responses immediately. Pay attention to your responses and report them to your Wellness Instructor. This helps us map out what direction your body is going. We've had some people cancer free in one month, and then again, others that have taken up to two years. Of course, how long the illness has been in your body, and how much damage has been done, will likely affect how long recovery takes.

Q: Can I work with The Divine Three Protocol and still do chemotherapy or radiation?
A: Absolutely. Although, with chemo, we know it is going to take longer to repair the damage created by this poison. Now with traditional X-Ray radiation treatments, we have found that when someone is going to partake in radiation treatments, and starts using the stones beforehand, they will almost always have a much easier time getting through the treatments. In other words, even though it is a different kind of radiation that the hospitals use, the stones still will acclimate the body to these man-altered energies.

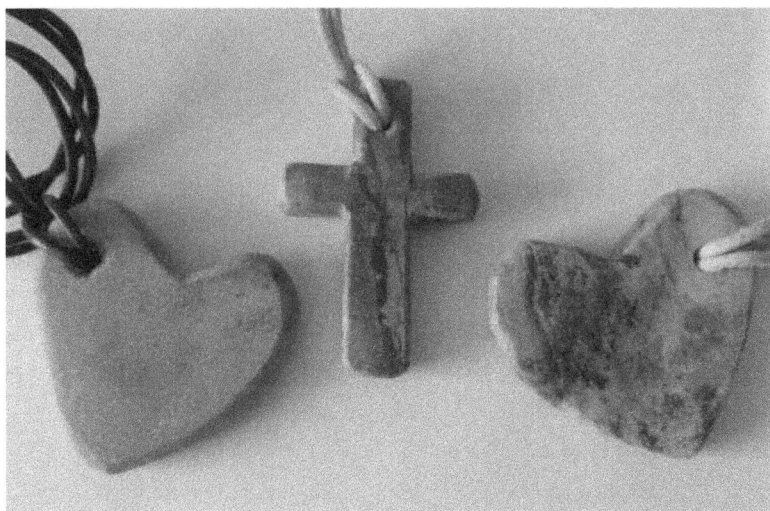

Q: What are the side effects of using radiation hormesis as clients begin to experience the toxins being eliminated because of using the stones?
A: There are side effects. It's a die off reaction. The side effects can be anything from "I just don't feel good" for a few days to headache, dizziness, nausea, achiness, fatigue, diarrhea. Jay and the

Wellness Instructors are watching closely because the client needs to acclimate to the radiation. If a person's system is very sensitive, they will need time to adjust and gradually increase the strength of the stones.

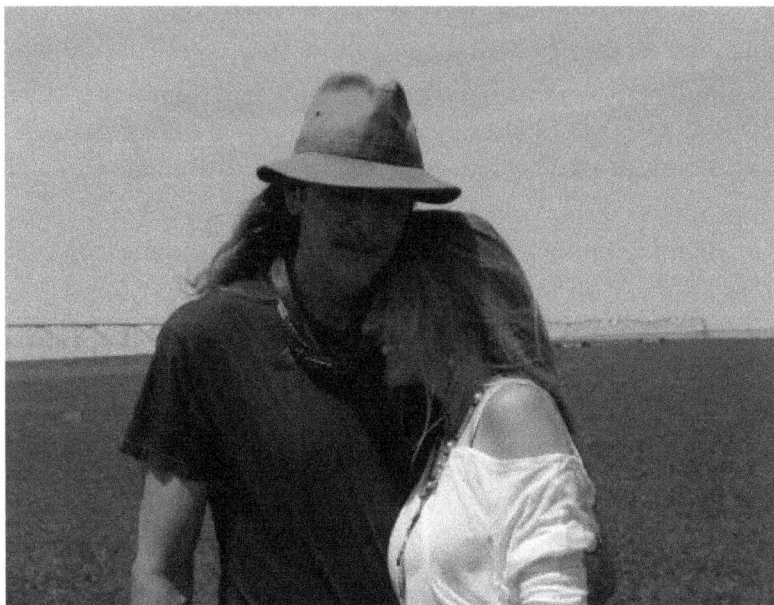

Q: I know I need to do parasite cleansing. I have the Water Divine Cleanse Kit and I have Dr. d'Angelo's parasite remedies. How should I get started?

A: The two days of intensive liver/colon and gall bladder cleansing opens up the bile ducts and removes toxic wastes. This allows the body to receive greater support in eliminating parasites. Remember to start with the Water Divine Foundation Kit minerals for optimal support through all of the cleanses and be consistent in following Dr. d'Angelo's remedies' instructions.

Q: Do I continue using the Water Divine Foundation Kit during the cleansing period—the 2 day intensive liver, colon, gall bladder cleansing?

A: Yes. These cleanses are for adults only. It is especially important to start using the Foundation Kit minerals 10 days prior to starting the liver/colon cleanse and during both the liver/colon and the gall bladder cleanses. This will help the body stay hydrated and may avoid possible leg cramping for those with magnesium and electrolyte deficiencies.

When you are going through the three month moon cycles of the parasite remedies prescribed by Dr. d'Angelo, it is important to also continue using the Water Divine Foundation Kit minerals during that time.

The only time to stop taking the Water Divine Foundation Kit minerals is when you take Copper in the Toxic Sludge Cleanse. For 10 days, while you are taking Copper, you stop taking all other minerals, so the Copper can do its job of eliminating parasites.

Q: In Dr. d'Angelo's parasite remedies protocol, what is the purpose of the Aroma Tab?

A: The Aroma Tab is a very natural, broad spectrum antibiotic made up of six essential oils. It is specifically targeted to patients who have yeast, so it would not be prescribed for someone with a parasite who does not have accompanying yeast overgrowth. The anti-yeast protocol is a combination of the Aroma Tab plus Silver. The side effects are minimal. In close to 4,000 patients, we have seen a 2 to 3 percent incidence of stomach upset.

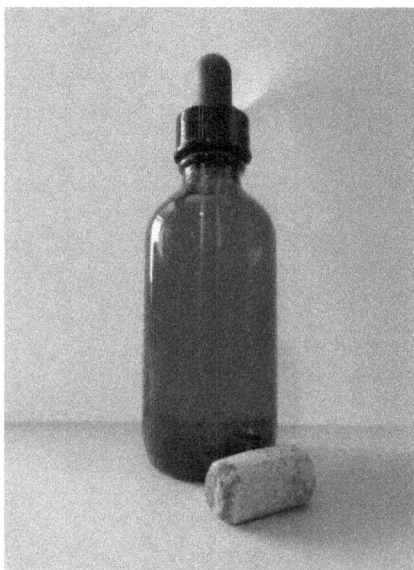

Q: How do the magnesium flakes fit into The Divine Three Protocol?

A: They are put into the water, for foot soaks and soaking in the hot stones hot tub. Magnesium soaks in through the skin. It is important in 300 physiological reactions, and is a critical component to generate energy in the human body. It also comes into play with the minerals that come from Walt and Kathy. That magnesium is in angstrom sized amounts, which guarantees that the magnesium will be absorbed internally.

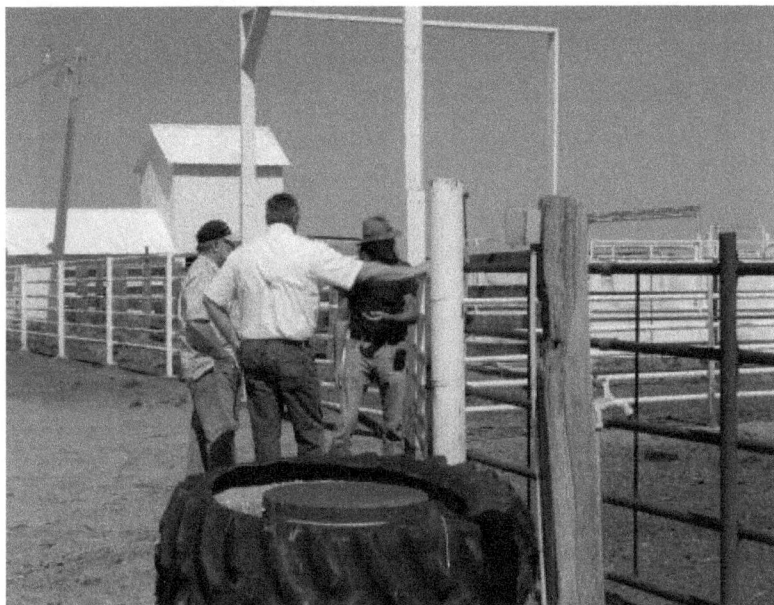

Q: I have read that sodium bicarbonate kills cancer cells. Should bicarbonate of soda be part of the protocol?

A: Cancers need acid to grow. They make acid as they destroy tissue. If you use more oxygen and more alkalinity, then you are working against the cancer. It is a valid protocol.

What we are finding is: if you put a hot rock in the water, it alkalinizes the water no matter what the pH is that you start with. It takes it to the right pH, so we are reformulating how we work with cancer wounds. We now know the frequency in the water is the right life-giving, healing frequency to use with any cancer.

Yes, you can use sodium bicarbonate externally. It will help. The problem is in taking it internally. The quantity of sodium in the sodium bicarbonate will overload the kidneys. So its much better to drink stone water.

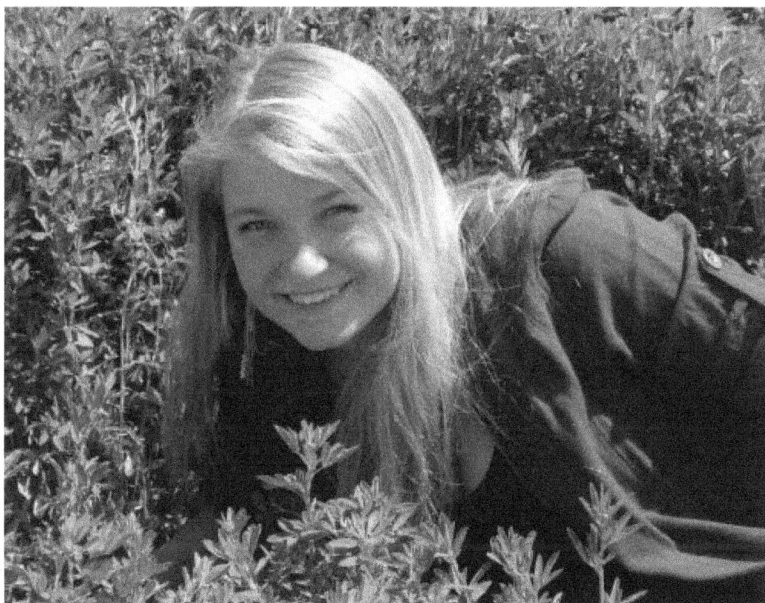

Vanessa Cox.

Q: Do I need to get the whole Radiation Hormesis Kit?
A: Every item in the Kit is a tool. With a half life of 250,000 years, it is like a first aid kit that never expires. I personally believe that every breathing person should own a Kit and a Grey Stone. Your Wellness Instructor will guide you on where, how long, and what steps to take. Even after we have cleared up the main health issue, whatever health problems arise, we can use these tools to help the

situation.

Q: Will using the stones interfere with the medications I am using or the supplements I take?

A: We have *never* had a conflict with using the stones that would complicate a health issue. As far as prescribed medications, we watch your body's responses to The Divine Three Protocol and work with your doctor to gradually reduce or eliminate the need for the medications.

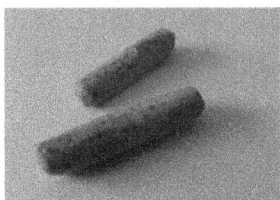

Q: Will the stones be enough, or would I go through the whole Divine Three Protocol?

A: We worked many years with clients using just the stones, but after traveling around the country, we learned that in many cases, more was needed. Through experience, and the guidance from God, we realized how vitally important it is to establish a system which is inclusive of all the elements, the minerals, and the vitamins required for the body to perform.

This was accomplished when Faye and Jay joined forces with Walt and Kathy Merriman, and Dr. d'Angelo and Nancy. Water Divine does work! Also, most healers and doctors around the world are always going after the yeast, or candida, that is, cancer. You will never get control of the candida/cancer, if you do not stop what is damaging the tissue: *parasites*.

The Divine Three Protocol is designed to obtain optimal health for even someone who supposedly has no health issues. Because of the cost effectiveness and support with this program, we all highly recommend this protocol to everyone from healthy to severely challenged.

5

TESTIMONIALS REGARDING THE DIVINE THREE PROTOCOL

W E HAVE ALL HEARD THE saying, "So often, life is what happens when you are busy making other plans." You read about some of these life stories in Chapter One. In this chapter Jay reflects on some of the stories which remind us that each life ultimately belongs to God, and is being divinely guided to a destiny we may or may not understand. We do all we can to support a person's intentions for healing and ultimately surrender to trusting that we are *all* in God's hands.

PART I
Donna S.'s story, as of April 2, 2012

> My name is Donna. Two years ago, October 2010, I felt a lump in my left breast. I was visiting grandchildren in Pennsylvania at the time, and was told it was a cyst. It kept growing. My husband and I thought it would be best to wait until we returned to Colorado to see my doctors. One is a chiropractor which I had been seeing for 9-plus years, and the other is Dr. d'Angelo, who had just

retired.

My chiropractor treated it as a cyst, but the lump
kept growing. By July of 2011, my nipple area had
started to change. I thought I should go get it
checked medically. I saw a nurse practitioner
where Dr. d'Angelo had worked. She sent me for
further tests which included ultra sounds,
mammograms, and biopsy testing.

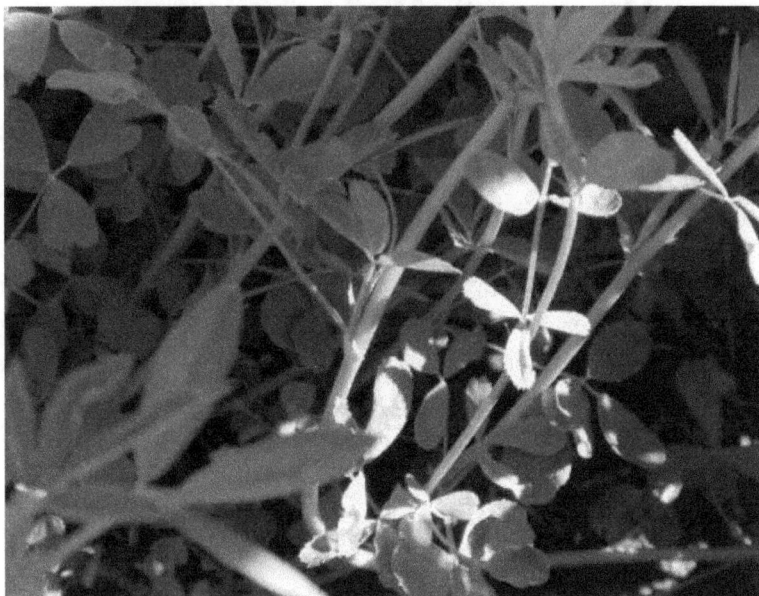

Two days after that diagnosis came, I got a text that
Dr. Raphael d'Angelo was holding a cancer
awareness class. So my husband and I signed up
and went to it, even though my husband was tired
from work that day. We decided to go and praise
the Lord that we did, because Dr. d'Angelo
introduced radiation hormesis to us that evening.

He pulled a rock out of his pocket, put it in my hands and said, "I think you need one of these."

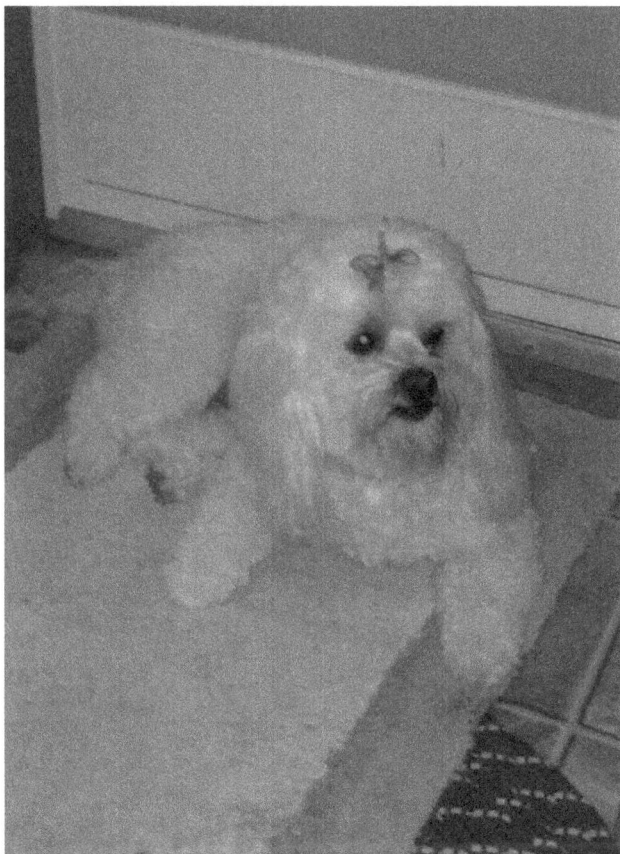

Logen has been on the radiation hormesis program since three months of age.

I was surprised to say the least! My worry and anxieties were building. I just did not want to do the expected chemotherapy and radiation the clinic doctor told me I would have to do. I was also told I needed a PET scan at the hospital because they wanted to see how far my cancer had gone.

By September, I was already on the radiation

hormesis (RH) rocks, using the Pendant, Mudpack, Hot Stone and Green Stone. In December, the PET scan revealed no cancer in my lymph nodes. The RH rocks were doing their job. It was working!

So I chose to heal my body the more natural way, which was the radiation hormesis frequencies (RHF) way. I started to wear the rocks faithfully, and changed my diet to more of an alkaline diet, like Dr. d'Angelo suggested. Then, I began losing weight and started feeling better. I did my parasite testing and started taking the Water Divine mineral water and now I am at the Mineral Palace because I want to be free of this challenge I have. Dr. d'Angelo and his wife, Nancy, and Faye and Jay have been helping me a lot. They keep me encouraged and tell me I am going to be O.K.

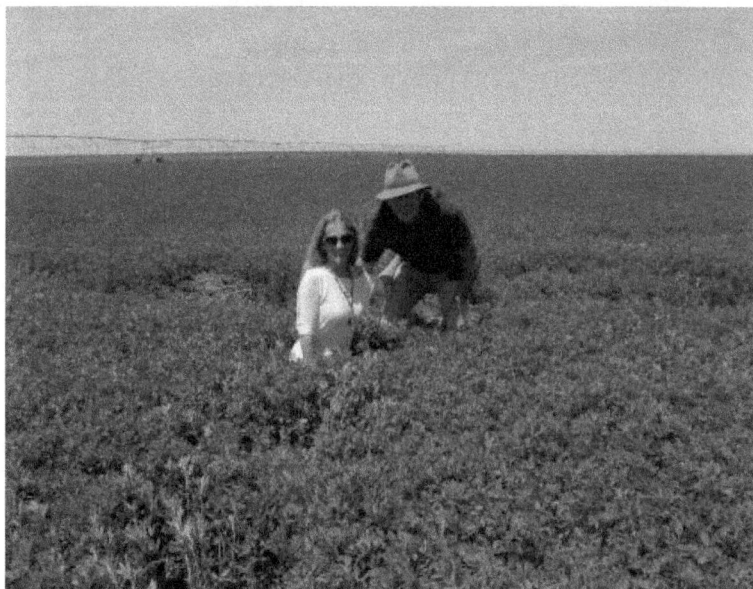

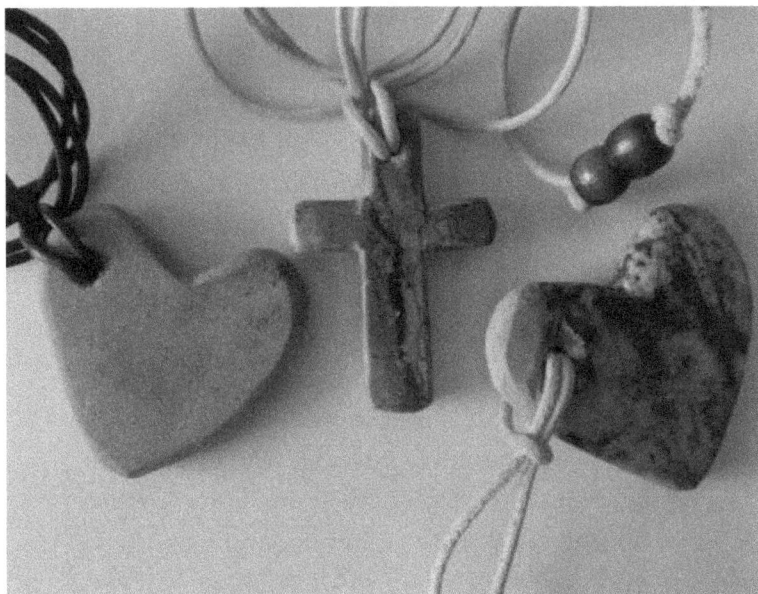

On March 19, 2012, I had a persistent cough and went to the doctor's office to get it checked. I received a call from Dr. d'Angelo after returning to the Mineral Palace for more RHF support. He told me that the newest X-ray showed I was now stage 4 breast cancer with nodules in the lungs. The prognosis was that I was in my final stages of life. With that news, Jay and I increased the RHF therapies.

On April 12, 2012, less than 3 weeks at the Mineral Palace, my cancer began to die off. The tumor was split and runny, which caused me to have an anxiety attack. Faye called Dr. d'Angelo and he said, "that is what happens when cancer starts to die off." I have been getting into the hot stones frequencies room, and the hot stones hot tub three times a day, here at the Mineral Palace, and I am now seeing positive changes.

Growing up in a Godly Christian home, I have a close personal relationship with the Lord. Since the cancer diagnosis, I claimed Jeremiah 33:3. It says, "Call unto me and I will answer thee and show thee great and mighty things, which thou knowest not." That verse has been an inspiration to me because cancer these days is a great and mighty thing. And the way they treat cancer is very deadly. I did not want to go that route, so I asked God to show me a different way. And, I called on Him and He is answering my prayers. And because I called on Him He is going to show me how great He is and what a Mighty God I serve.

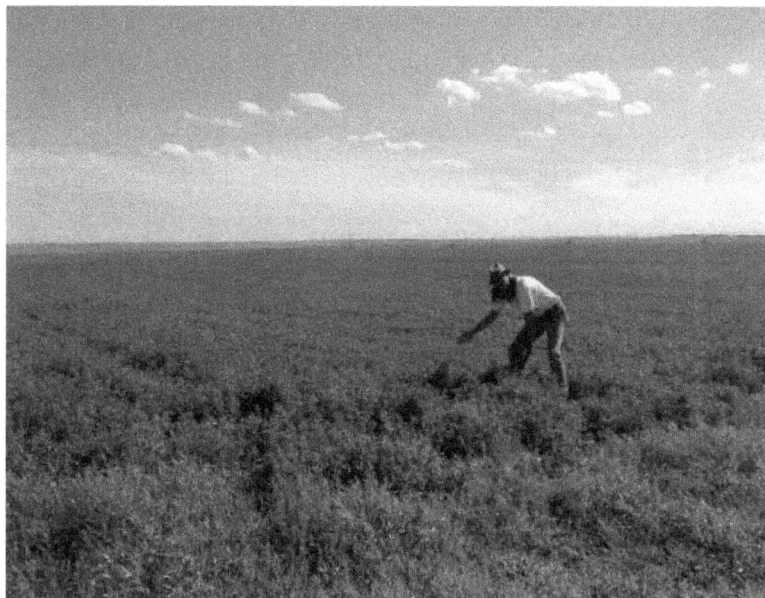

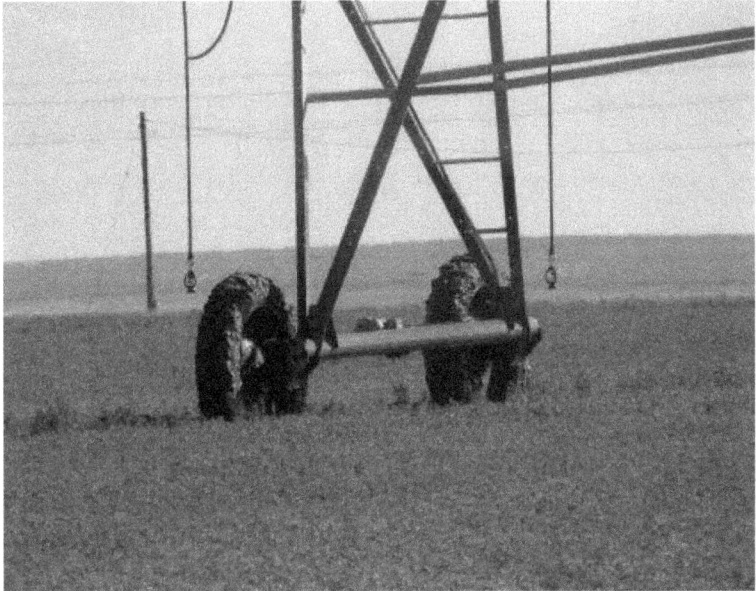

Question: What has been your response to the Water Divine minerals?

> I started taking the Water Divine minerals when I first came in February of 2012. I spent the whole weekend here at the Mineral Palace with Dr. d'Angelo and his wife, Nancy. I have been feeling a lot stronger, a lot more energetic. I have not been "sick" since my cancer diagnosis. I have been feeling healthy other than the fact that I have bronchitis right now.
>
> I feel great. I feel energized. I feel renewed. So many mornings I wake up and think, I cannot believe I have cancer until I look at my breast. That is my constant reminder.

Question: What has been your response to Dr. d'Angelo's

parasitology?

> I started parasite testing in November. At that
> point we were not sure the rocks were going to
> work, so we thought if we get rid of the parasites,
> we should be pretty close to being cancer free.
> Round worms, protozoa and candida are what he
> found. He put me on Formula PZ and Formula
> MZ. He added Silver and Aroma Tabs/Essential
> Oils. Later, he took me off the Silver and Aroma

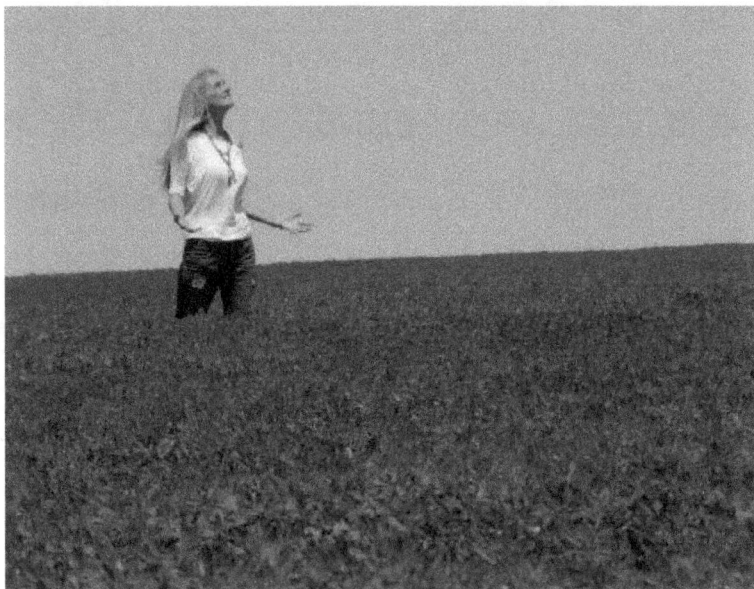

Tabs and I am still on the Formulas PZ and MZ.

> I do see a difference now. When I would think
> about my cancer, I would get nervous a lot. I
> would have to use the bathroom often and have
> diarrhea. He said, "that's a sign of parasites." It

settled down since the parasite cleanse. I have been doing the parasite cleansing along with the Water Divine Foundation Minerals, and consistent exposure to the RH Frequencies. They are now starting to break up the tumor.

Question: What has family support been like?

My family support has been from my parents, sister and her husband. My sister's husband lost his sister to leukemia 5 years ago. He saw what chemo did to his sister, so he told me to stick with this protocol. He did not want me to go through what his sister endured. My sister said she probably would have done the chemotherapy because she's not patient enough to do what I am doing. Still, she encourages me and assures me I have chosen the right path.

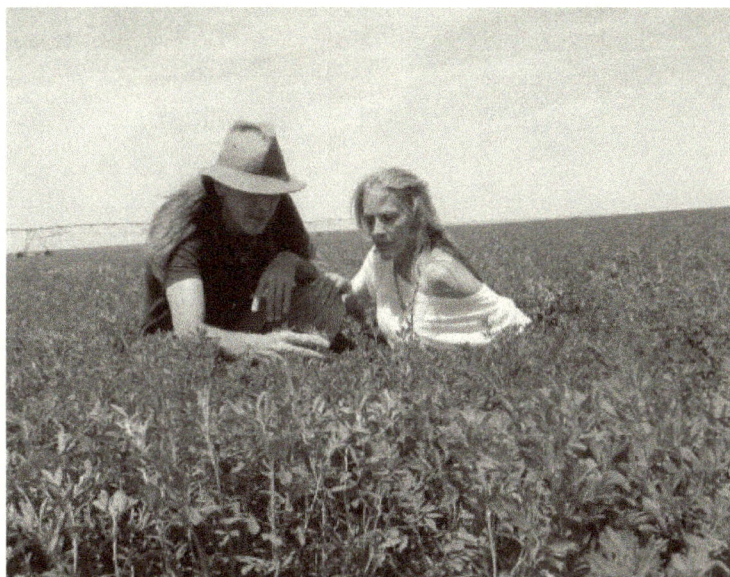

My parents have been supportive since day one. They believed that once I was in Dr. d'Angelo's care, I would be alright, because I have a good physician watching over me.

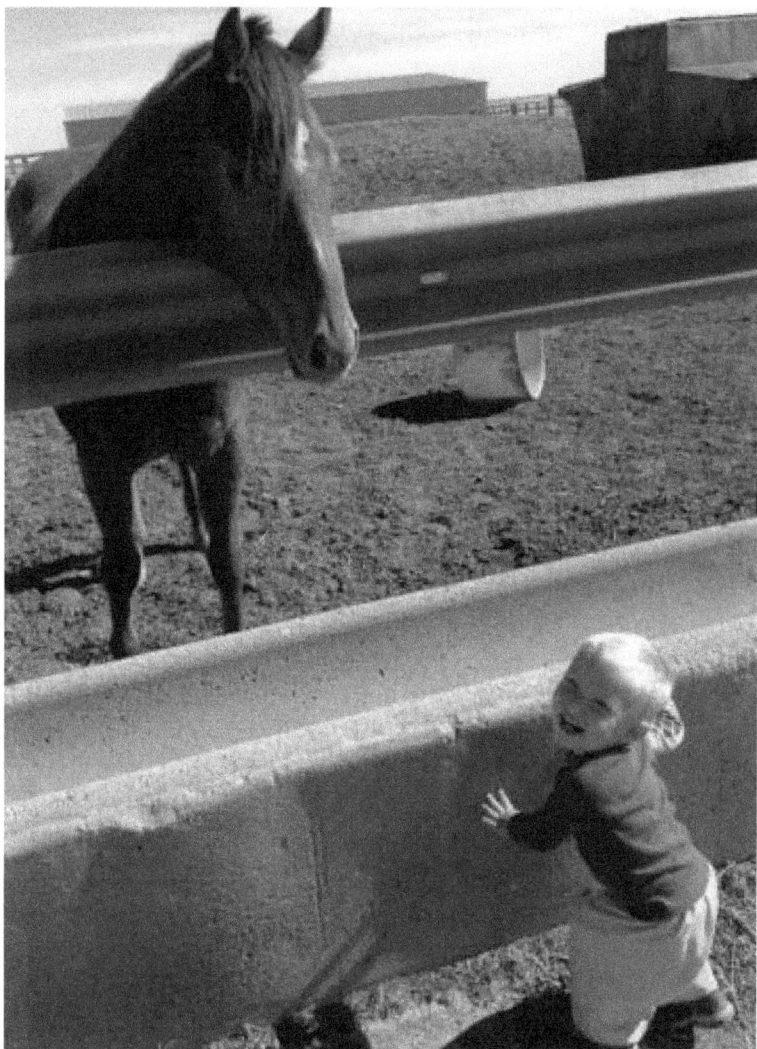

Emmett Cox and friend.

My husband has been a rock. I get teary when I talk about him because he was the one who told me I had cancer. I could not take any more phone calls from the doctors because, at that point, I just did not want to have any more bad news. He called the doctor that night and as we were getting ready for dinner, I asked him if the doctor called. He nodded yes and started to cry. Then I knew I had cancer. He said the doctor said it was stage 3 breast cancer. He is a very wonderful man and has been by my side every day since the diagnosis. I am blessed to have a wonderful husband. Today he called and cried and said he misses me. So I said, "I miss you too. Please don't cry."

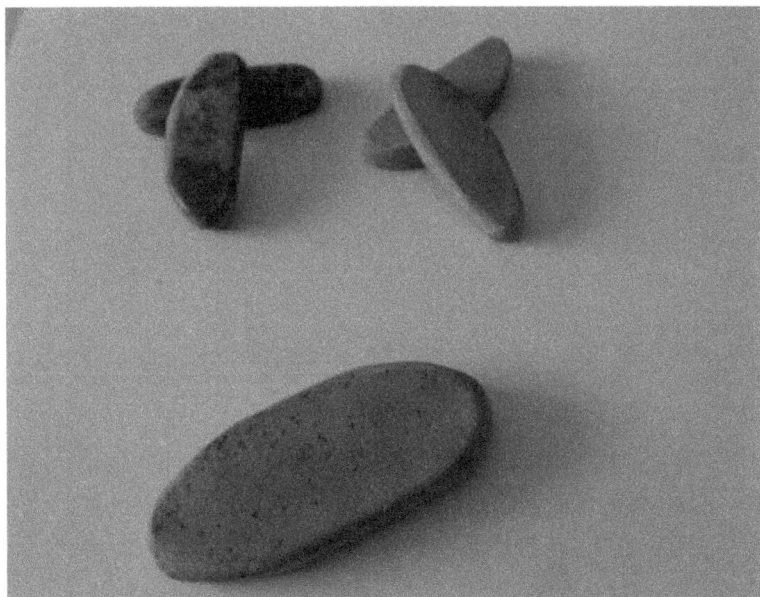

We have 3 children. Our oldest daughter, at first, was for me doing this naturally, until she heard that the other doctors had told me it had spread to my lungs. Then it scared her, and she wanted me to do the chemo. I told her I wasn't going to and her response was, "Oh Mom, we love you." She's scared. I know she sees me doing OK and she wants to be supportive. My son knows I have cancer but he doesn't choose to share his feelings about the path we've chosen. Nor does he have anything to do with me.

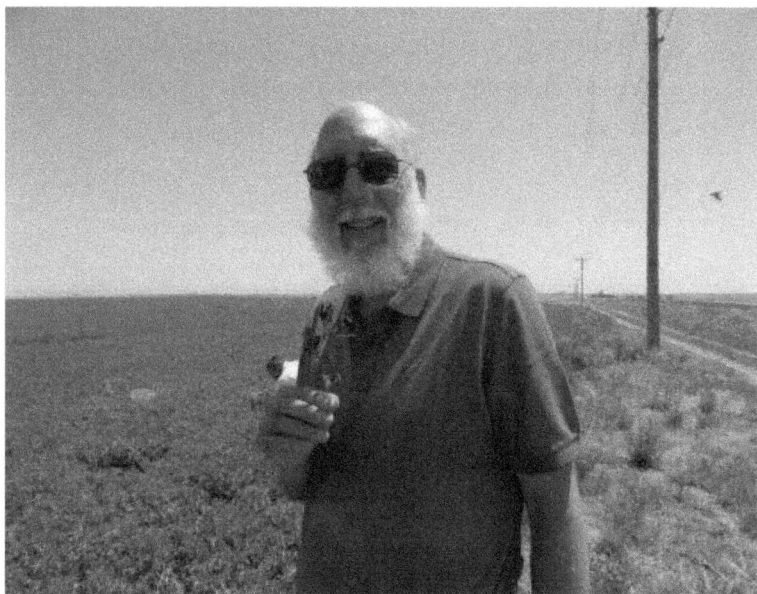

Our youngest daughter would feel better if I had chosen the chemo way. She has friends whose family members are in the medical field, and have influenced her that chemotherapy is *the* way to be treated. As of right now, my treatments would have been 6 weeks of chemo and 3 weeks of radiation.

I have stage 3 breast cancer. It was also labeled grade 3, which means it was the aggressive form of cancer. Grade 3 is 50 to 75. Mine was at a 53. They had me take antibiotics for 4 weeks, and the antibiotics were really flaring up those parasites. I remember telling the doctors that certain parts of my body were itching because of the parasites and the doctors said that sometimes the antibiotics can do that.

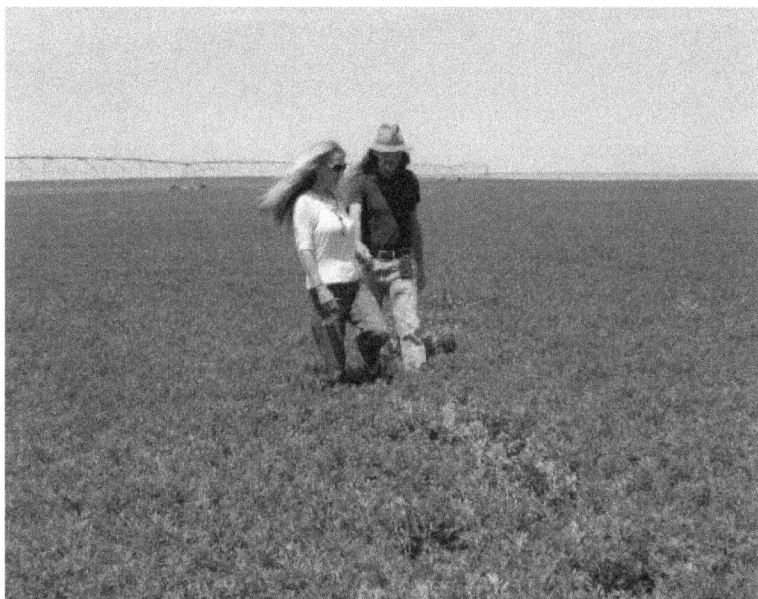

Now I realize the antibiotics made the parasites mad. The antibiotics flared up the parasites and made them more aggressive. If I had not taken a whole month's worth of antibiotics, I do not think it would have developed into a grade 3. Only God knows that.

I serve a mighty God. He knows what my next journey will be and He is not done with me yet. I know that because I'm getting better and I am getting stronger, and as I said before, I have never really been sick since this whole thing started, anyway. Here I am today at the Mineral Palace and I am determined to stay here until it is gone.

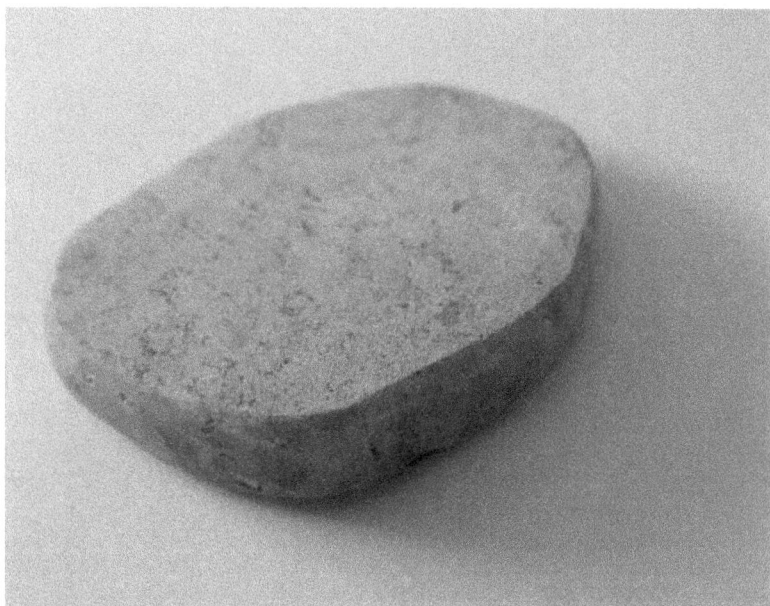

Having this lump in my breast for over a year, I am tired of it. I want it to end. I want to sleep on my stomach again and exercise. I want my life back! I do not want it to take over me, so that is why I am here. I had asked Daniel, my Wellness Instructor, how long will it take to get rid of it? He said, "How long do you want it to take? 30 days, 60 days, 90 days?" I said 30 days would be wonderful. He said, "Well you're going to have to stay here until its done.

Right then, the lightbulb went on. So I went to
Faye and said I'm staying. I am done with this. I
will stay until it's gone.

Question: If you were talking to a woman with breast cancer
similar to yours what would you say to her?

I would say, I know you are scared. You are very
scared. Because I was scared. If you have 30 days,
I would mark the calendar and get here as fast as
you can because you have to get acclimated to the
levels of natural radiation. Once you get
acclimated, then you know your body is accepting
all of those life-giving, healing frequencies and you
know you are on your road to recovery.

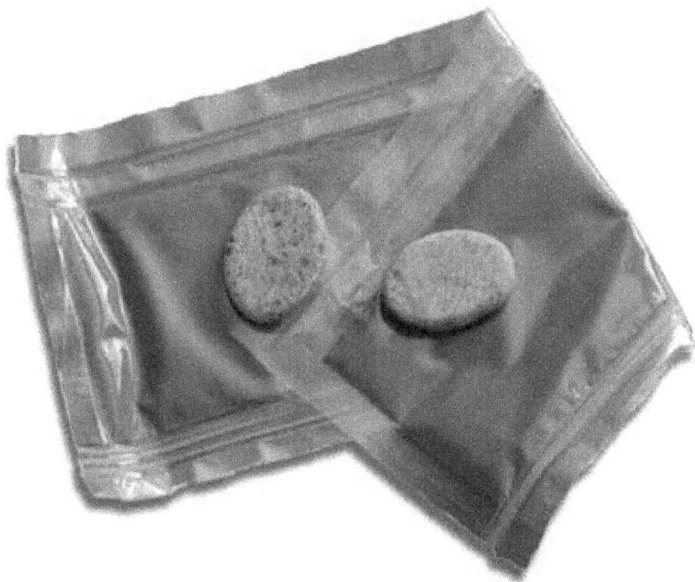

At first when I came down, I thought I was going to be healed in 4 days. I thought, OK, I am going to get in that tub and wear the rocks 24/7 and sleep with the Mudpacks. After 4 days it was still there.

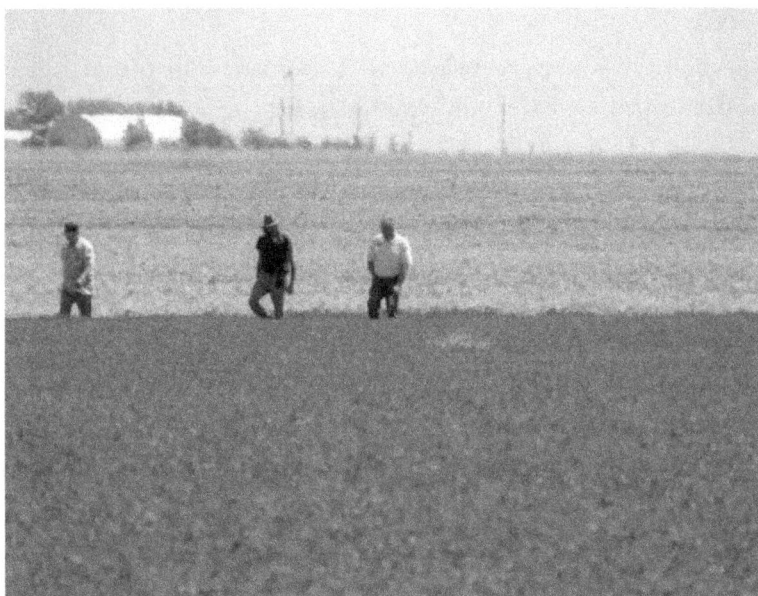

I do not know how long I have had my cancer. I could have had it for 7 or even 10 years. It is going to take a while for it to be gone. It was foolish of me to believe it could be healed in 4 days. During the three weeks here so far, my breast opened up and the tumor started coming out. So I have a big open sore. It has started to heal now. It was ugly and it still is ugly, but it is going to be alright. Once the healing started, I saw the cancer begin to leave my body.

I am a student too, so I bring my school work with me and I stay busy. The routine they have me in always keeps me busy. So I would say get here when you can. It is worth it!

If you are afraid, turn to God. He is there 24/7. He is always there, even if you think He is not. He is always listening. He will always be your closest friend. Then find the support you need through your family, your closest friends, and you will get great support here at the Mineral Palace. Just get here!

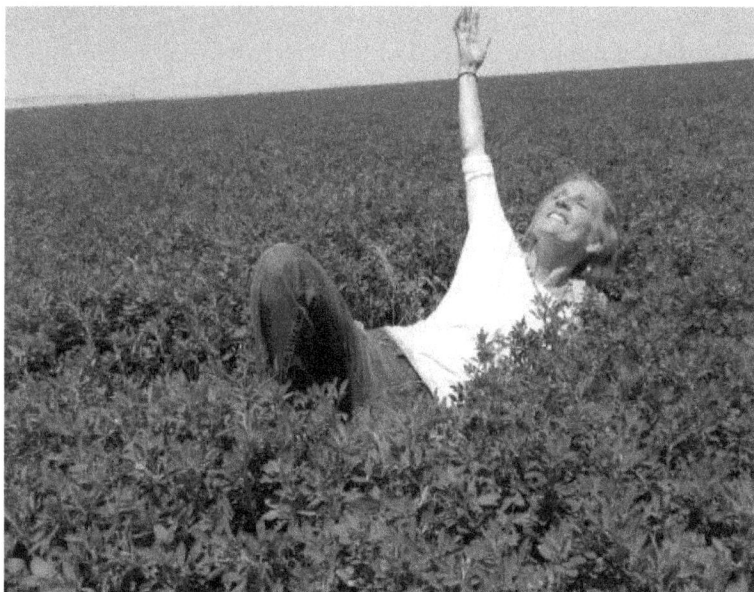

Wellness Instructor Report on Donna as of 5/19/2012:

After watching Donna's commitment and dedication to The Divine Three Protocol, we have been astounded at her progress, and were able to observe the process work better than expected. Once we introduced the frequencies to the tumor, we witnessed her body orchestrate an elimination of the mass and repair of the wound. The love and support from her family, especially her husband Phil, has been critical to her success. Donna should be considered a role model for anyone who is battling a disease.

Mack's story, told by Wellness Instructor, Jay Gutierrez, on April 27, 2012

> Here at Night Hawk Minerals' Mineral Palace, we have been blessed to witness many miracles. We thought it would be important to tell Mack's story.
>
> Mack has been a friend of the family for years. He is 51 years old, and was sent to us by family members in Iowa. Mack is from way back in the hills and has little formal education. That never stopped him from learning how to take a Jaguar engine apart and put it back together in pristine condition.

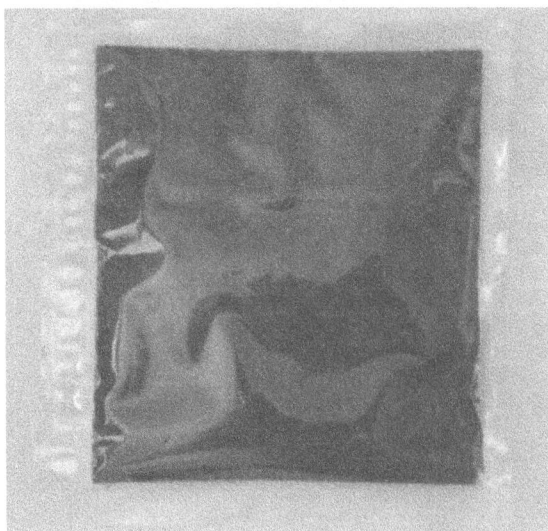

Mudpack.

When he came to us 5 months ago, in January, his heart was dying. His doctors had told him, 8 months before he came here, that he only had 9 months to live. He actually had a card in his back pocket that explained where to send the body!

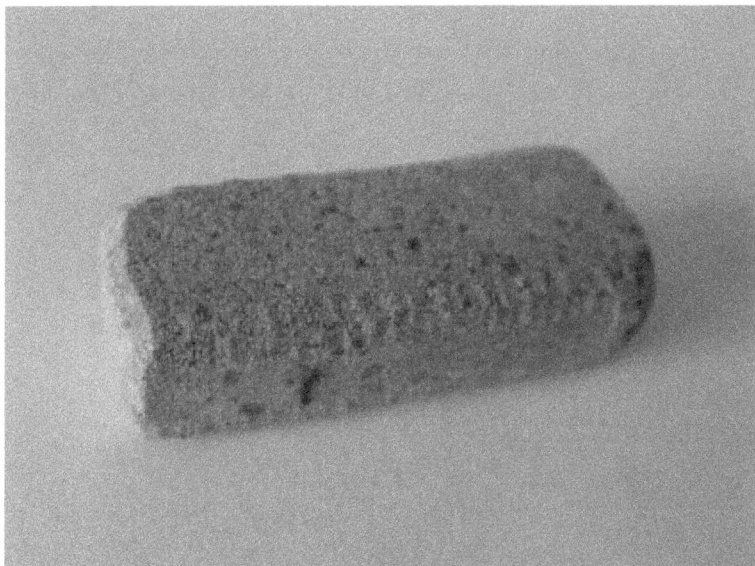

When he arrived, he could hardly walk three steps before being out of breath and needing to rest. We immediately put him on The Divine Three Protocol. This meant he got help from Dr. d'Angelo and his wife Nancy, and he started taking the minerals from Walt and Kathy at Water Divine. Walt had suggested that along with the Foundation Minerals we were giving him, that we should put him on what he calls a cardiovascular cocktail.

The first week Mack was here, we would put him in our tub at the Mineral Palace which contains uranium ore, large raw pieces of chrysocolla, and magnesium chloride. We also had him parasite tested, and we monitored his diet. He slept all day, every other day.

The next week he was able to do therapies every day. We saw dramatic improvement in his health over the next 3 weeks. By the time he left here, he was working on cars, and had done so well, we sent him home.

His doctors in Iowa were in awe and have reported that over 50 percent of his heart had *grown back*!

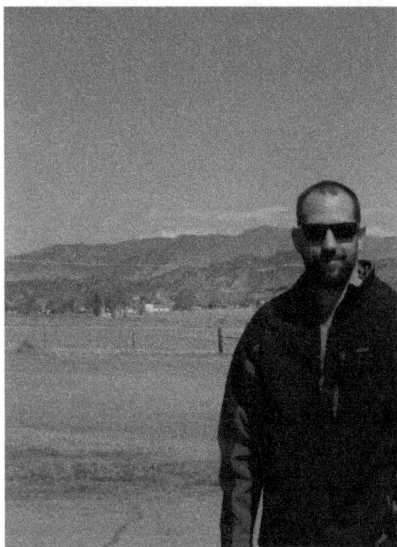

Daniel Cox.

Wellness Instructor Report as of 5/19/2012:
Mack is home now and doing great. He has remodeled his home and is back to work. We were his last hope. Even though here at Night Hawk Minerals, we work mostly with cancer, we have had experience with many degenerative diseases with great success. I personally feel that what makes these kinds of testimonials such a blessing, is that they have all been explainable with what we have learned over the years. Mack will return every six months or so for a visit, but at home he has been faithful to following the protocol with his stones and has been given a second chance. — Jay Gutierrez

Stories of Trela N. and Charlotte F., told on May 22, 2012

Trela and Charlotte have lived together in Pritchett, Colorado, for almost eight years. At 92 years of age, mom Trela has a sharp mind and quick wit, though her body now needs the support of a wheel chair. Trela and her husband raised eight children. Charlotte, the middle daughter, is now 67 years young. She and her husband raised two children and the extended families are now scattered between Colorado, Utah, Nebraska and Wyoming.

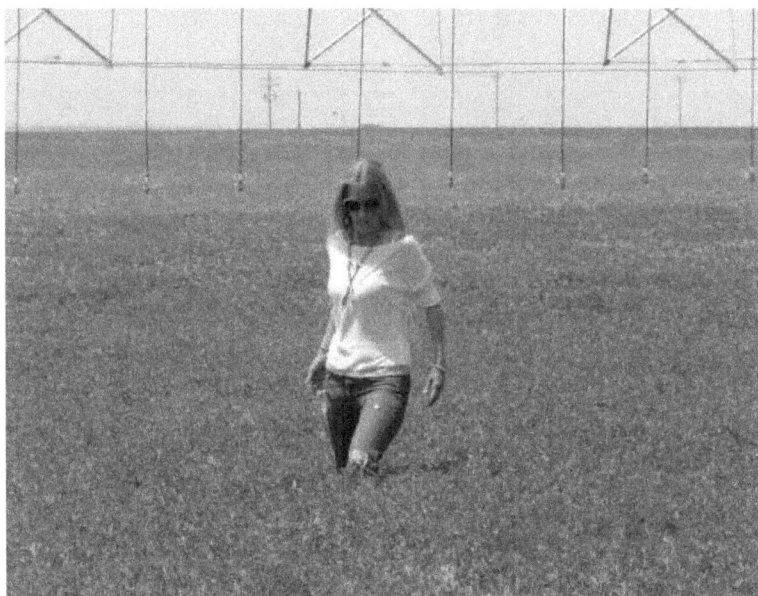

Both Trela and Charlotte have had transformational healing experiences with the RH rocks, which Faye and Jay brought to their community in the spring of 2008. Their stories are told here, in their own words.

Trela's Story:

    The first time I saw them was when they came here

and held a meeting for the whole community. There were many of us who went to the meeting, the building was full. They showed us the rocks and told us what they were doing. After the meeting I went up to Jay and told him I had lumps in my breasts and didn't know what to do about it. Jay gave me a Kit and told me how to start wearing the stones. I started using them and before I knew it, within a few months, the lumps started disappearing and finally went away. And I was so thrilled about that! They're still gone!

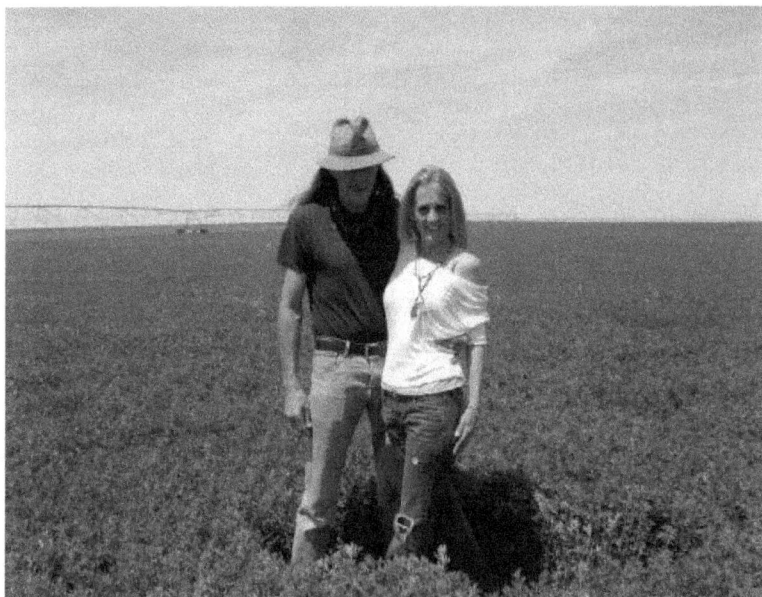

Now I still use the stones in my bra, and I wear the mudpacks on my knees. They take the pain away. I'm feeling so thankful that they came along with the solution. I have never heard tell of such a thing as these rocks and the Kits. They have a lot to do

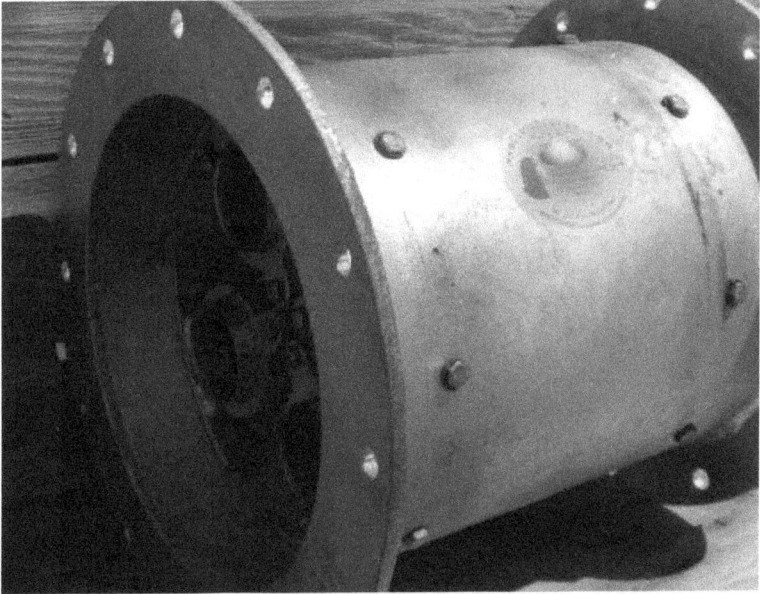

with why I'm still here doing so well!

One other concern I have is a sore on the side of my nose. It never goes away, so we had it checked—skin scrapings sent to a lab in Denver—and it is a form of skin cancer. Dr. d'Angelo said to use frankincense every night and every morning. So we added that to the protocol and now it looks much better, like it's going away.

Charlotte's Story:

When Jay and Faye first came and held the big meeting, in 2008, I didn't have much the matter with me, that I knew about. I did get a Kit and used their rocks. By 2010, when they came together and opened up the Mineral Palace, I had started having health problems. In the spring of

2010, I went to the doctor and was just feeling really bad. At that point, I could only get through half a day, and then I was done. So my doctor sent me to a liver specialist in Salt Lake who said I had cirrhosis of the liver. The liver was swollen and the bile ducts were closed. The most common causes—drugs and alcohol—weren't anything I had ever done, so they couldn't explain why I had such a bad liver.

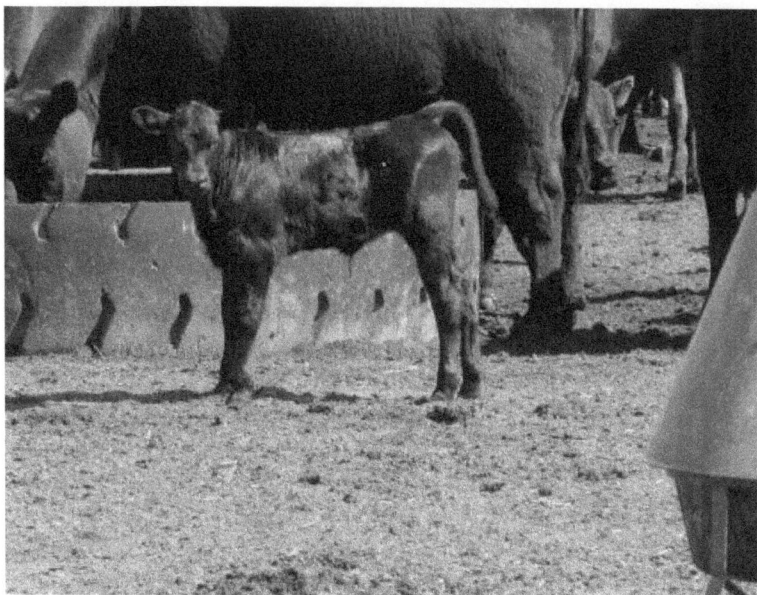

Then they checked my blood and said I had Polycythemia Vera, which is a form of leukemia. Polycythemia vera is a bone marrow disease that leads to an abnormal increase in the number of blood cells—primarily red blood cells. They wanted me to start taking some chemo pills.

That's when I called Jay. He told me to not take

the pills, but to come down and get on the protocol. I remember the words he said to me when he saw me, that meant so much. He said, "Charlotte, we're here to help you, and more than that, we'll fix you!" So I started with three things: getting into the hot stones hot tub, the ozone sauna, and ozone directly on the liver. I did these three things twice a day for ten days, after the specialist had run an ultrasound on my liver. After those ten days, I went back to the specialist for an MRI. It showed that the liver was functioning properly at that time. It was still enlarged with swelling, yet the bile ducts were open. The ozone had opened up the bile ducts, and got the blood flowing.

After that doctor visit, I kept saying "no" to the chemo pills and went back to Jay and Faye, and the

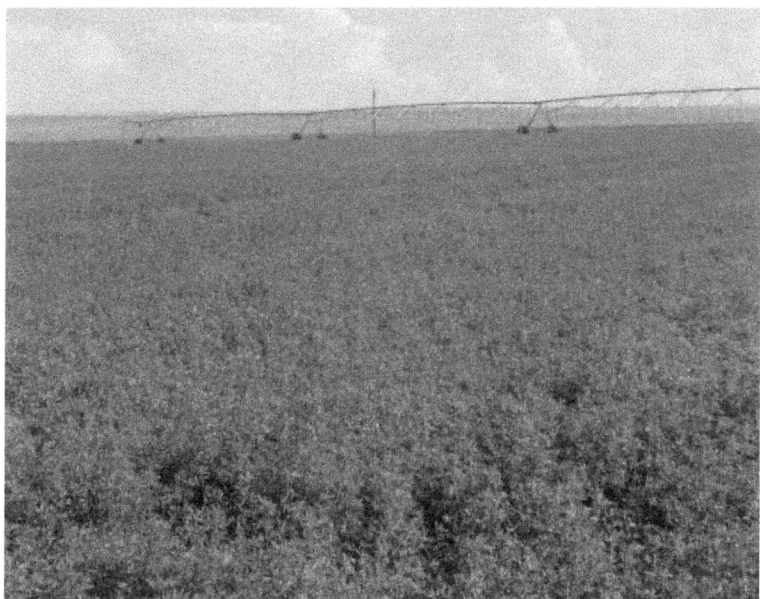

protocol. At that point, Jay got to checking for parasites. He had done enough research to learn that some of these parasites are linked to people's health problems.

> Jay and Dr. Hammed Ibraheem checked me for parasites and I had two of the worst parasites—*Ascaris lumbricoides* or round worms, which come from dirt, and *Heterodera radiciola*—a very common root-parasitic nematode that grows in a great variety of plants, including root vegetables as radishes, celery, carrots, and potatoes.

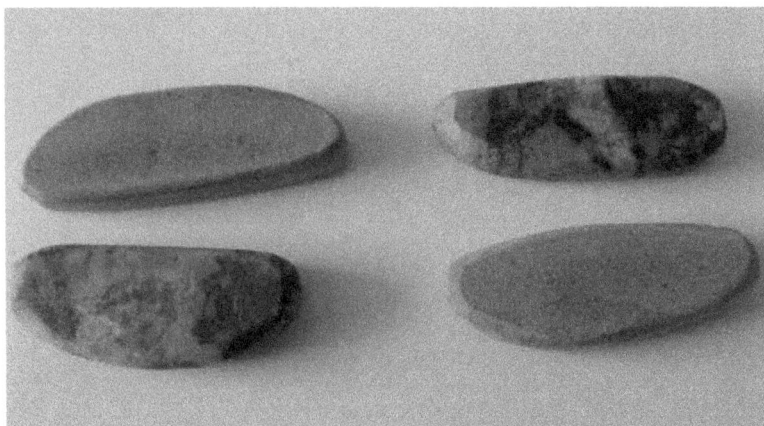

> The first round of remedies came from Dr. Ibraheem in Nigeria. While I went through that protocol, Jay and Dr. d'Angelo teamed up to make the process more accessible and more affordable. So I went through Dr. d'Angelo's parasite cleanse protocol for eight to nine months. Because the parasites were in all stages—fully grown, larvae, and eggs—we had to go after them in the ways they cycle according to the moon cycles. One of them

had gone up the bile duct, from the intestine, into the liver and was causing havoc. The parasites were so resistant, I had to go through the remedies for two more cycles, each one being stronger than the one before, until we cleaned them out. Finally, the tests showed that I was rid of parasites. The blood counts—the white blood cell count, the platelet count, the red blood cell count—were all abnormal, showing they were all too high, all through this time.

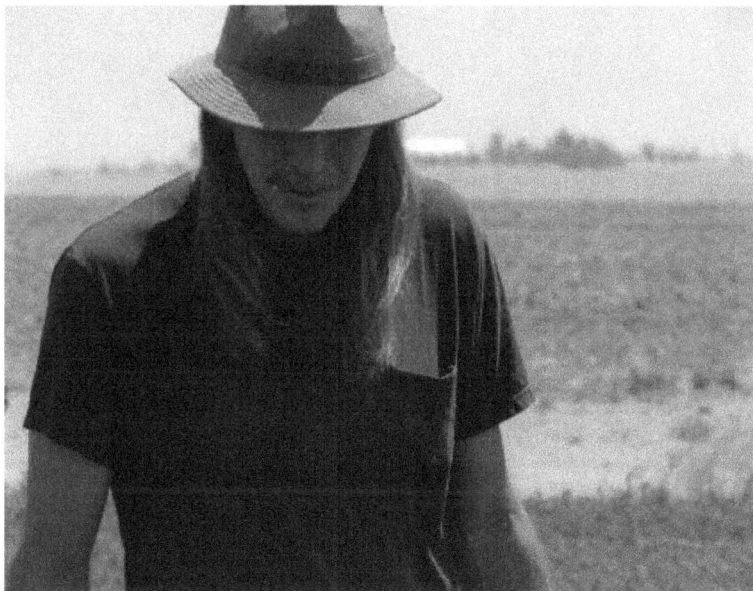

So after we got rid of the parasites, and I stayed on this protocol, faithfully, for over two years, my white blood cell count went into the normal range. It was during this time that I added the third part of The Divine Three Protocol. I started drinking the Foundation Minerals Kit water from Water Divine, and I went through Water Divine's liver/colon cleanse and the gall bladder cleanse. My liver was clean, but lots of stones appeared on the gall bladder cleanse.

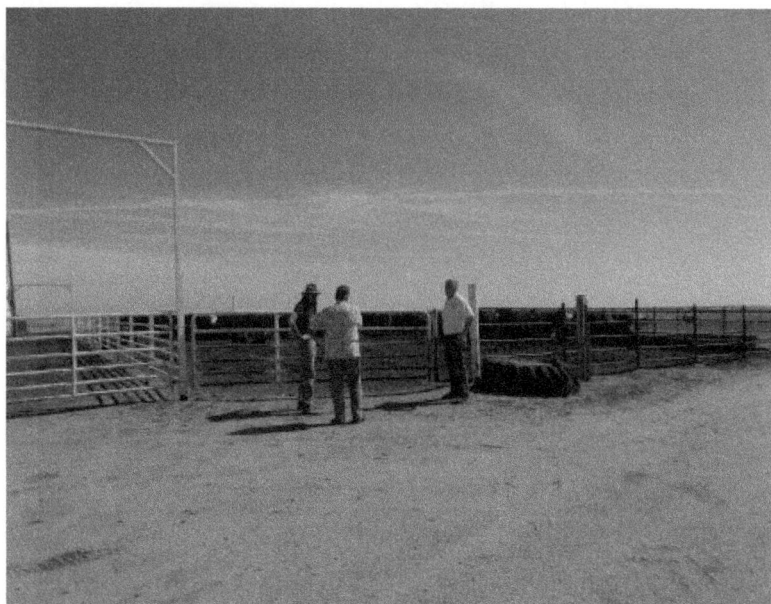

I also completed two more of the seven cleanses recommended by Walt Merriman. I drank ½ oz. of angstrom-sized water-soluble Copper each day for 10 days. After a week off, to let new eggs hatch, I drank the copper again, except this time I added zinc, which helps the copper go after the parasites in the harder to reach places. This was called the Toxic Sludge Cleanse. I finished off the cleanses with the Immune System Cleanse. For 10 days, I took angstrom-sized, water-soluble Silver.

During this time, while I was completing the

cleanses, my blood counts remained normal. The Water Divine part of the protocol really helped build me back up and I started feeling like my old self again, with plenty of stamina and energy to get through the day.

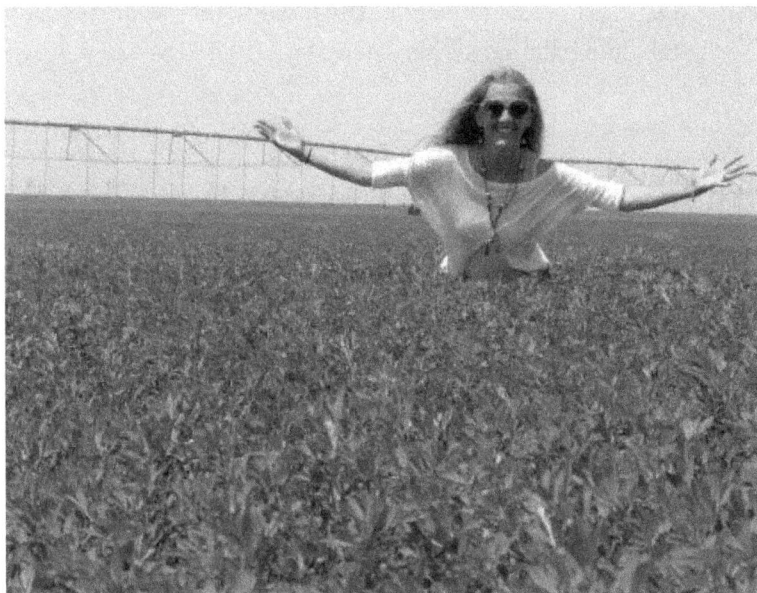

It's now the end of May, 2012. Using each part of The Divine Three Protocol, all of my blood counts went into the normal range and continue to be completely normal. I just went back to the doctor and had my two year check up. The liver is now back to its normal size. There's still some scarring, likely from hepatitis I had when I was in college. They told me that some of the damage of the liver probably came from that. The parasites are gone and my immune system seems to be handling what it needs to take care of, so that I feel strong and healthy again.

To give myself optimal support, I sleep on the bigger sized, body mud-pack, and I also put the rocks and the smaller Mudpacks on my knees. It takes the pain away. I also have the formulas from Dr. d'Angelo and Nancy which work very well to take the pain out of my knees.

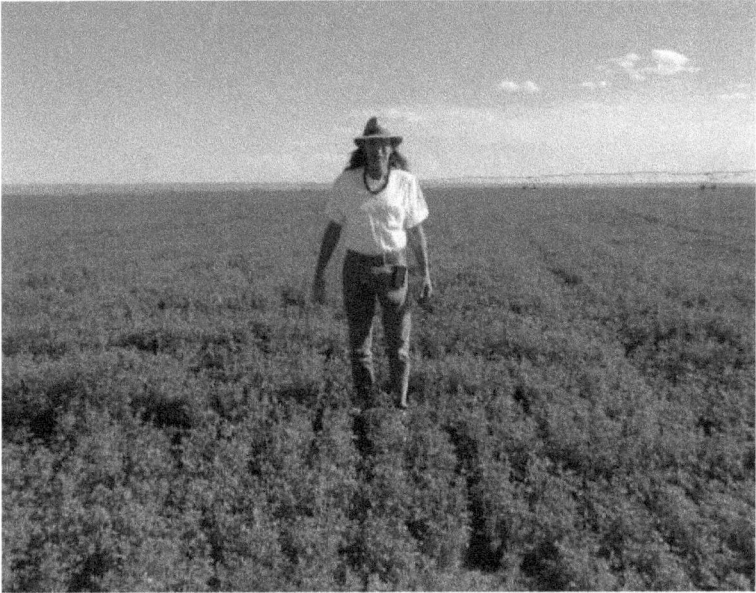

Question: Regarding family support, have the members of your family helped you to work with The Divine Three Protocol?

The family has watched. At first they were not sure this would work. They said, "if it works on you, then we'll believe it!" They really did not think the hot tub and the rocks and all the other parts of the protocol would stop the cancer. Now that they have seen it work, there are several of them who have started using the products.

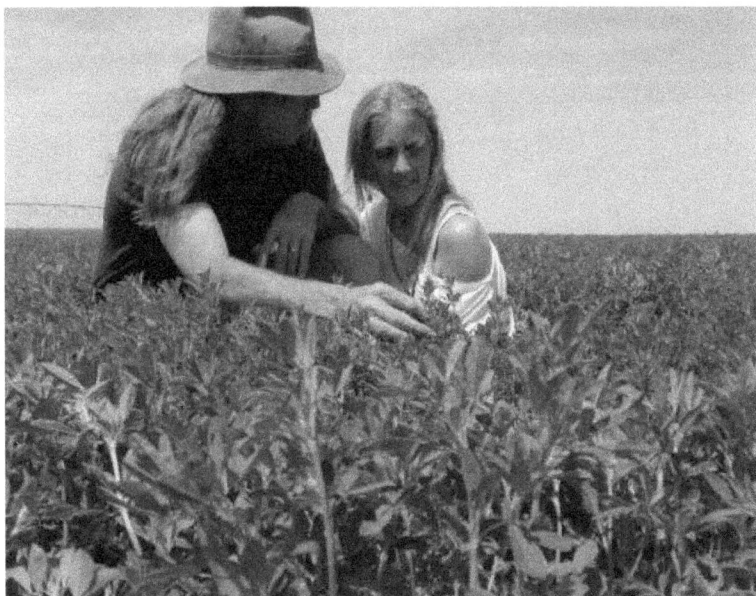

My brother, Jerry, not only went through a round of The Divine Three Protocol for himself, he and Jay had already put the hot stones in the drinking water for his cattle. They set that up in 2009. Jerry says it makes the cows want to drink more water and after watching them for more than two years, he says they stay healthier, especially the calves! He also said the water in the tank stays clear and doesn't grow the algae which used to make the water mossy.

Question: If you knew someone with similar issues, what would you say to them?

I would tell them to get here and get on The Divine

Three Protocol, and don't quit. Expect it to be an up and down battle because there are times when the mind will say, "Is this really working?" There are days when you feel really really bad and you get scared. So you have to have some trust for Jay and Faye and the Wellness Instructors and let their support and encouragement get you through the down days. Just stay with it and you will get it whipped.

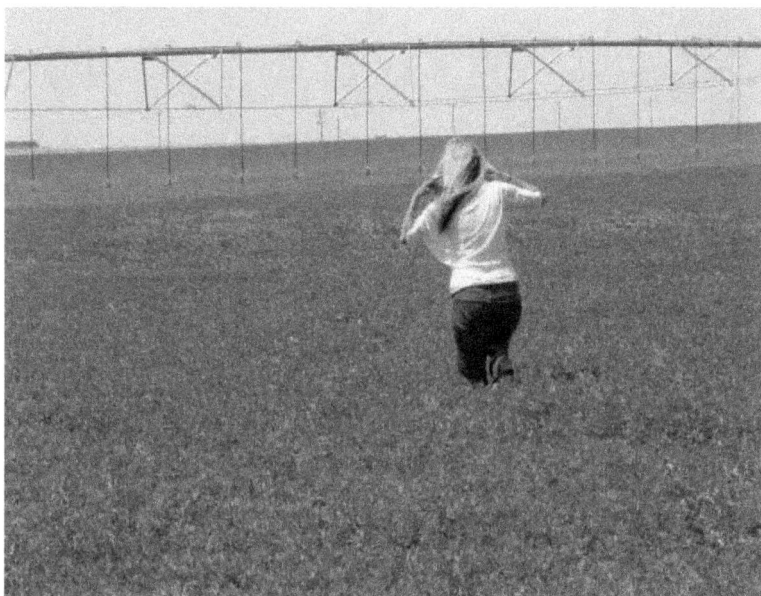

And, anyone with allergies, or sinus and lung problems will be helped with the inhales, breathing the steamy RH Frequency water from boiling the bigger green and hot stones. So I would encourage them, whatever they've got, to get down here with their problems and go through The Divine Three Protocol. I know, from my own experience, it will help. If they don't wait until it's too late, they will get help, and they will get better.

Question: Is there anything in your religious beliefs that brings you into conflict about using The Divine Three Protocol?

No, I was a Christian before, so it has not affected my faith in any way. I do believe that a person has to believe in the protocol they are using, and stick with it, for it to have a chance to work.

WELLNESS INSTRUCTOR REPORT AS OF 5/19/2012:
When Faye and I first came to this small town, we gave a presentation. In the back was a lovely older woman who came to me at the end of the lecture and said, "I have lumps in my breasts and I don't know what to do about it.

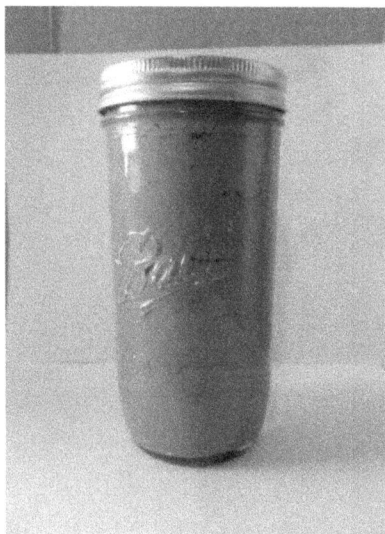

Faye and I decided to gift this kind lady a Kit and breast stones. We did not hear from her for a while. After we moved here to Pritchett, we found out the woman also lives here and her lumps were gone! She is in her 90's now and still using the stones. We love Trela.

Charlotte's strong will and being proactive in conquering leukemia was admirable to say the least. She said, "I'm not going to do that dang chemo, fix me!" We did. Charlotte has also been an incredible support for others that pass through our doors. Many thanks go out to Charlotte for being a big part of discovering answers that helped put The Divine Three Protocol together. She will always be family. — Jay Gutierrez

JIM D.'S STORY: SAVING THE HONEY BEES FROM COLONY COLLAPSE DISORDER, REPORTED IN MAY, 2012
According to the Natural Resources Defense Council (NRDC), honey bees are disappearing across the country, putting $15 billion worth of fruits, nuts and vegetables at risk.[2] Beekeepers first sounded the alarm in 2006. Seemingly, healthy bees were abandoning the hives en masse, never to return. Researchers call the mass disappearance "Colony Collapse Disorder," and they estimate that nearly one-third of all honey bee colonies in the country have vanished.

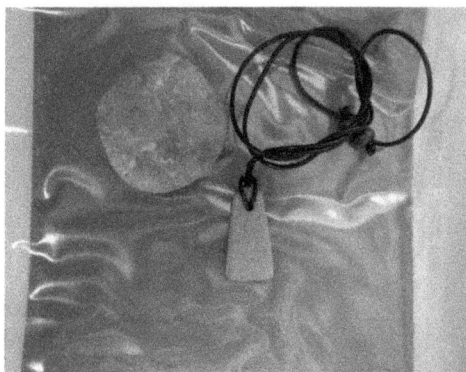

Why? Scientists studying the disorder believe a combination of factors could be making bees sick, including pesticide exposure, invasive parasitic mites, an inadequate food supply and a new virus that targets bees' immune systems.

What can be done? In the next 5 years, the USDA has allotted $20 million for research. At the same time, the potential loss is expected to be $15 billion worth of crops that bees pollinate every year. No honey bees will mean no more apples, cucumbers, broccoli, onions, pumpkins, carrots, avocados, or almonds. The

2. Website: www.nrdc.org/wildlife/animals/bees.aspgclid=CK3E-6znrrACFWrptgodZxTRUg

list includes at least 42 known fruits, vegetables, and field crops, not to mention the flowers.

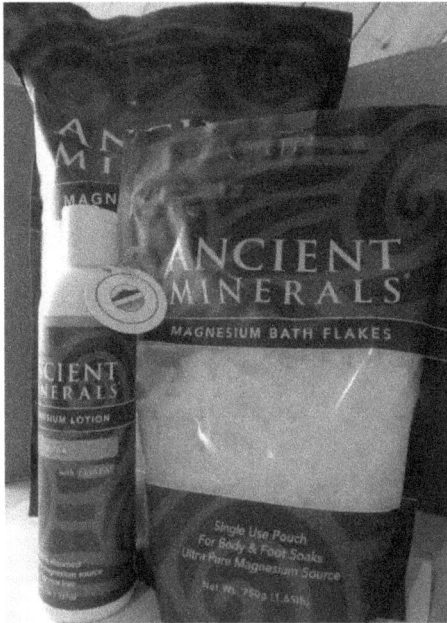

Beginning in early March of 2012, as a result of the experiments that Jim and his beekeeper friend, Ray, have been doing, putting Jay Gutierrez's "hot rocks" in the sugar water, next to the honey bees' hives, they have a story to tell about what will save the honey bees from disappearing. Jim and Ray live with their families in the Virginia Piedmont, forty miles from the Blue Ridge Mountains, in a little town named Louisa. They are surrounded by the bigger cities of Richmond, Charlottesville, and Fredericksburg.

Jim learned about Jay's radiation hormesis frequencies from a neighbor who has cancer. Jim called Jay, and divine intervention took on a whole new meaning.

Jim reports:

> Jay said that I was the first one to realize it is not the radiation in the rocks. It is the harmonics, or the frequencies, that solve the problems. The radiation in the rocks is nothing more than battery cells powering the frequencies.

Jim's friend, beekeeper Ray, at that point, had two hives. After talking with Jay, Jim asked Ray to consider feeding one hive of his honey bees the stone water and leaving one as a "control." No one knew what would happen. Ray's response to Jim was, "I haven't had a single hive to last past three years before colony collapse set in. These bees are going to die anyway. I've really got nothing to lose." So the experiment was on!

Jim says:

> The first thing we noticed was the bees were drinking half again more sugar water than we had seen before. And then we noticed that the jars of water didn't need to be washed like they had before, because there was no growth of algae in the water like before. It also became obvious that the bees, which had been docile, who were now drinking the rock water, started working.

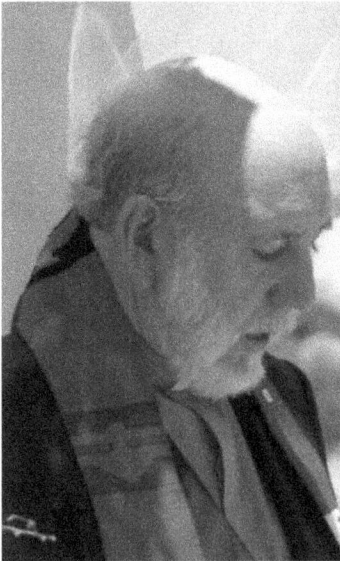

What happened next was something Ray and Jim had never seen before. The bees became more active and were working harder than any bees they had ever seen. What Ray knows about bees is that when they swarm, the new queen and her brood workers are left in the old hive and the old queen and her workers swarm out to go find a new home.

As a seasoned beekeeper, when Ray saw this happen the first time, he said it looked like the biggest swarm he had ever seen—at least 6 gallons of bees were in that swarm. So now, he had the old hive and a new hive, with some exceptionally hard working bees.

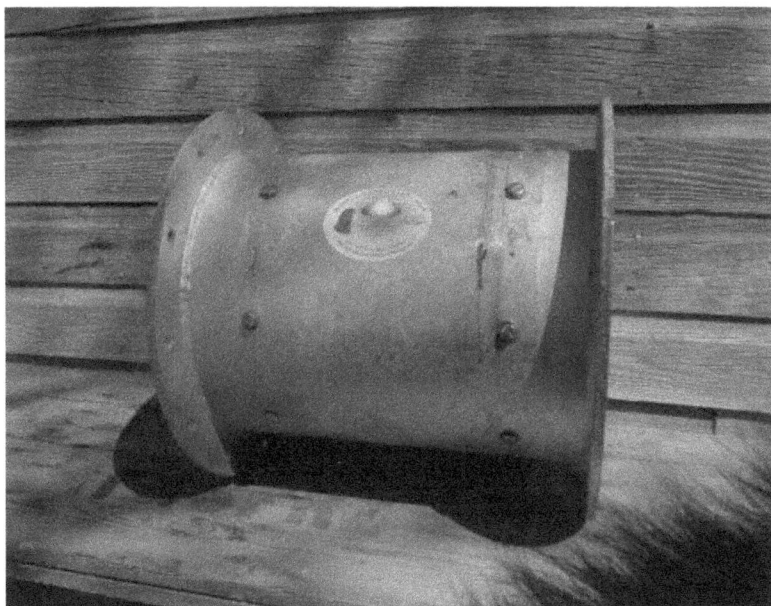

More amazing than that, within three weeks, the original hive had its second swarm, and within another four days, a third swarm came out with at least 2 to 3 gallons of bees. By this time, the original hive of bees had made about 50 pounds of honey. In less than two months, one hive of bees had turned into four and the bees continued to be the hardest working bees Ray had ever seen.

In the past, when bad weather would set in, the bees would become less active and just hang around the hive. These bees seem to have so much energy, they just keep working. Ray says they are by far the most aggressive bees he has ever worked with. "They will aggressively push other bees out of the blossom to go after the nectar. There is no sign of colony collapse, in fact, it is just the opposite."

Jim says he would be happy to talk with anyone who wants to know more about how they are saving the honey bees from colony collapse disorder. Call Jay first, and he will put you in touch with Jim. Jay's contact information is on the Contact Information page of this manual.

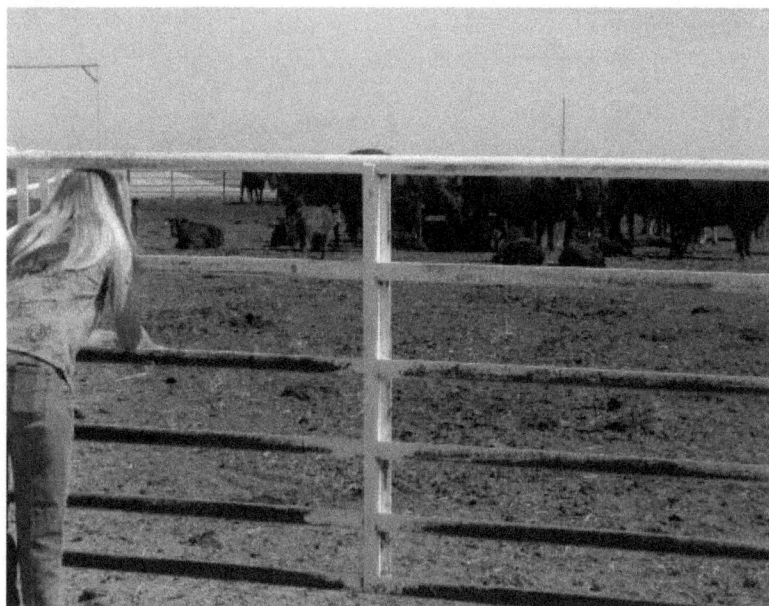

WELLNESS INSTRUCTOR REPORT ON SAVING THE HONEY BEES PROJECT AS OF JUNE, 2012

Once we proved the hot stones produced "life-giving frequencies," we realized that these frequencies imprint on what they come in contact with. When we put the hot rock in the sugar water, the frequencies imprinted the water molecules, which then kept on imprinting all the other water molecules in the sugar water. We knew we were introducing the correct life-giving energy to the hive.

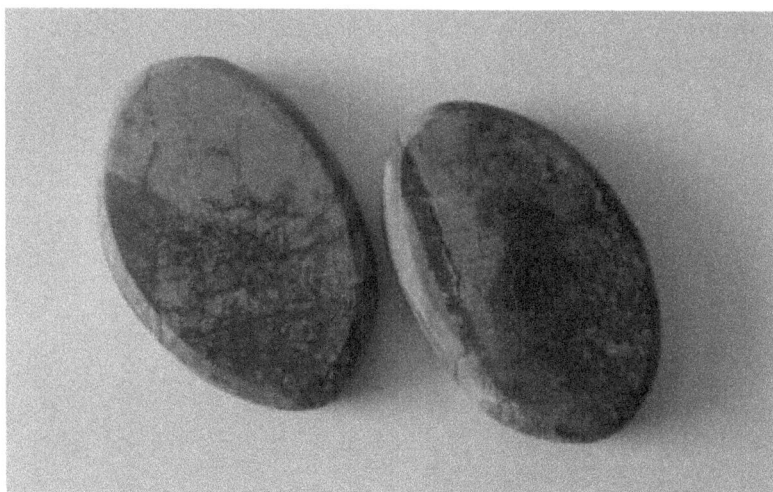

We also knew the problem with colony collapse disorder is an interruption in their system that facilitates communication and navigation. As we see it, because of the electromagnetic frequencies (EMF's), pesticides, etc., these creatures are going out to forage and get lost. It's like flying a helicopter without any communication and/or broken navigation equipment. It doesn't work.

What we have realized after working with these frequencies for some time, is that they will *always do the right thing*, and it always will eventually overpower a disruptive frequency or shatter toxic molecular structures.

The great thing about working with this energy is that now we know it *is*: the frequencies! They always have the effect we intended them to have. And most often, as with the saving of the bees, they exceed our predictions!

What we did is basically reintroduce the correct life-giving frequencies back to the hive and it naturally started producing at peak levels. I would like to thank Jim and Ray for stepping up to the plate and getting this information out. It takes courage to step out of the box, but these men have an overabundance of common sense.

I believe that these stones are God's Breath and can do no wrong.
— Jay Gutierrez

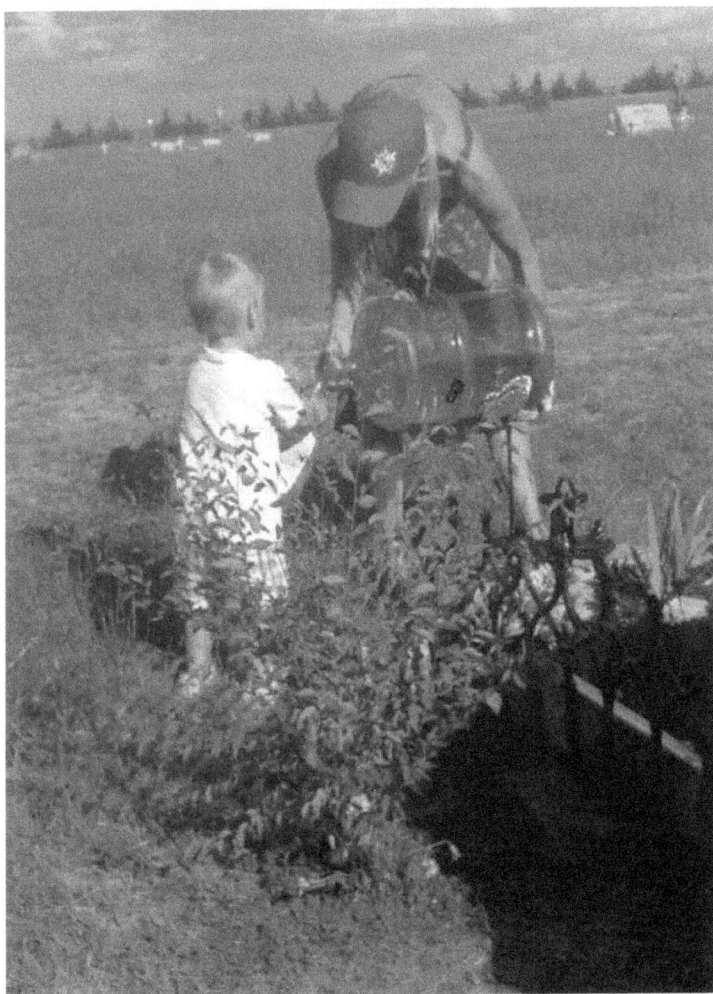

Emmett and Faye watering plants with structured water.

6

HONORED PATRONS

O VER THE YEARS WE HAVE learned incredible amounts of information pertaining to saving lives from these degenerative life-destroying diseases. Along this journey, we have had the honor of working with very, very special people who did not recover from their health crisis.

We are all family here at Night Hawk Minerals and would like to pay tribute to those who helped us make tremendous strides in learning. From understanding the importance of parasite testing, to holding their hand after finding out that they had too much chemotherapy and there was no turning back.

We are presently, as I see it, the most effective and successful protocol out there, and most of this was made possible from the ultimate sacrifice from those we remember. The legacy they left us has given many others a positive prognosis for their life. We will often remember these heroes, reflect on their teachings to help others, and forever honor their spirit. God Bless. Jay Gutierrez

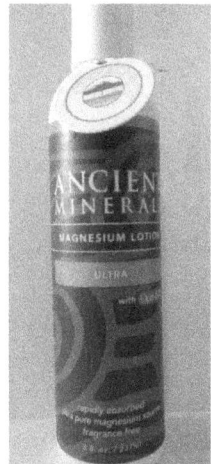

7

SUSTAINABILITY: PHYSICAL, MENTAL, SPIRITUAL ASPECTS

IN THIS CHAPTER WE WILL cover the following.

Factors: Important factors which allow the state of healing being accessed through The Divine Three Protocol to become a lasting state of balance, health, and well being.

Choices: Creating lifestyle choices to achieve the highest potential of living one's purpose and to enjoy life.

Resources: For nutrition, physical exercise, mental and spiritual attunements to living "in the positive."

Support: The Volunteer Servers Program.

IMPORTANT FACTORS
In addition to the myriad of colds, flu, chicken pox, and/or other short term illnesses we experienced as children, some of us have already, or are now facing life threatening degenerative diseases. Illness must be addressed on all levels: physical, mental, emotional and spiritual. Make sure your game plan for recovery includes

paying close attention to each aspect. Under "Resources" in this chapter, an excellent center to explore for addressing each of these aspects is AmazingLifeInstitute.org.

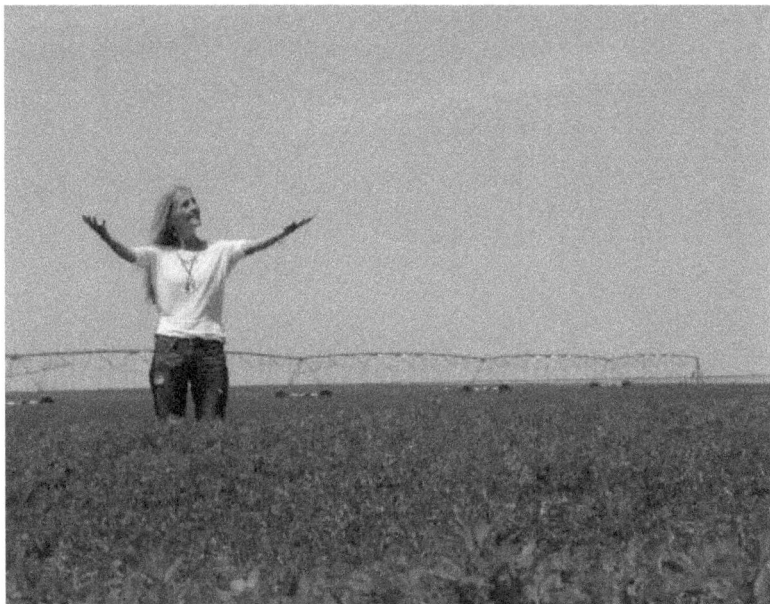

Regarding the treatments for illnesses, this manual presents a comprehensive plan in The Divine Three Protocol to address the issues causing problems: the parasites, the too-acidic or too-alkaline environment, the lack of oxygen, the deadly bacteria, mold, the tumors, the damaged cells, the missing minerals and nutrients the cells need to do their jobs, and the suppressed or overwhelmed immune system. The Divine Three Protocol, in most people, allows the shift to take place giving the body's immune system the boost it needs to bring the body back into balance and into a state of improved health and wellness.

Unless God presents a greater plan, if you commit to The Divine Three Protocol, you most often will begin to see results which will answer your prayers. You'll find some of these inspiring stories in Chapter 5.

There are also reminders throughout this book, humbling us to realize each life has its own destiny. We do all we can to support a person's intentions and ultimately surrender to trusting that we are all in God's hands.

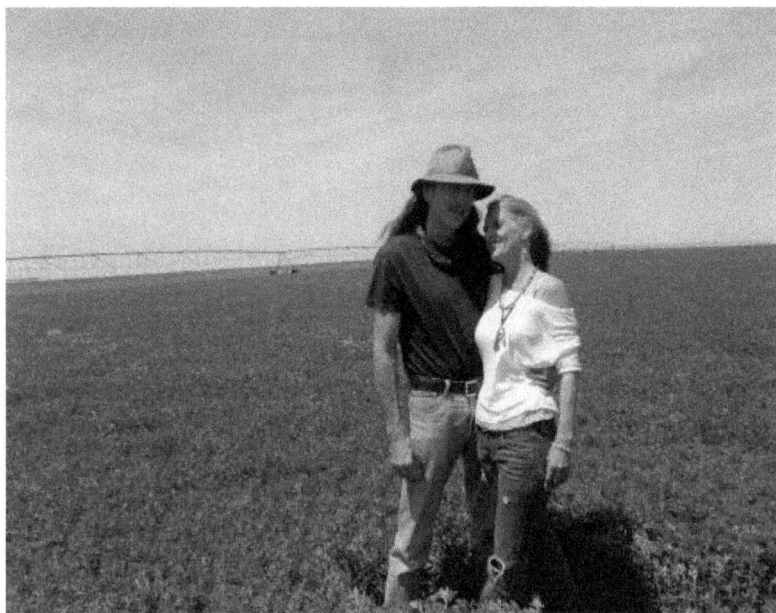

How will you sustain the state of health and wellness which The Divine Three Protocol brings to your life? You will gain such knowledge and wisdom as you go through the healing process. One factor is to share what you learned. Because of the depth of your understanding, in a heart beat, in some situations, you could make a significant difference in someone else's life.

A second factor is learning to enjoy being yourself. There's a satisfaction and joy that comes from the depths of your soul, because you "get your life back." In all of the 7+ billion people on planet earth, there isn't another soul, another consciousness, another heartbeat that can be or replace you. Working with the factor of being yourself, this is an important time to get in touch with your own thoughts and feelings about who you are, what you want your life to be about, and the choices you are making, to allow for the highest potential for living your life's purpose.

A very helpful exercise is to get a journal and begin exploring these questions and answers:

◆ Who am I?
◆ What does it mean to become more and more "myself?"
◆ What do I want my life to be about from this point on?
◆ What is my purpose/mission/calling?
◆ What is the gift I was meant to give?
◆ What must happen for me to fulfill this purpose?
◆ What changes need to take place within me to get in alignment to accomplish my purpose?
◆ What help will I need?
◆ What/who do I have to forgive in order to free myself to attract and receive this support?
◆ What out-of-my-control longings, which leave me feeling defeated and un-seen, un-heard, and un-wanted, do I have to surrender to God, to allow God to provide the Highest Good in a much larger picture of my life?
◆ What help will I need to move into the life God is patiently, with unconditional love, waiting for me to choose?
◆ What would God have me choose?
◆ When will I take the first, or the next, step?

Perhaps the greatest factor is your intention to love. We're told from many sources that there is no power greater than the power of love. Love heals. In the same way that Jay and Faye talk about the life-giving frequencies of radiation hormesis stones, the life-giving vibrational frequencies of love nourish and heal the body, mind, and spirit. If you withhold love from yourself, you interfere with your body's ability to heal. If you carry thoughts and feelings of separation—fear, hurt, anger, resentment—toward those who make up the world you live in, you separate yourself from love, and that too, interferes with your body's ability to receive the nourishment and healing energy of love.

Another factor is surrounding yourself with loving supportive family and friends, keeping the nay sayers and criticizers out of your energy field.

CREATING LIFESTYLE CHOICES

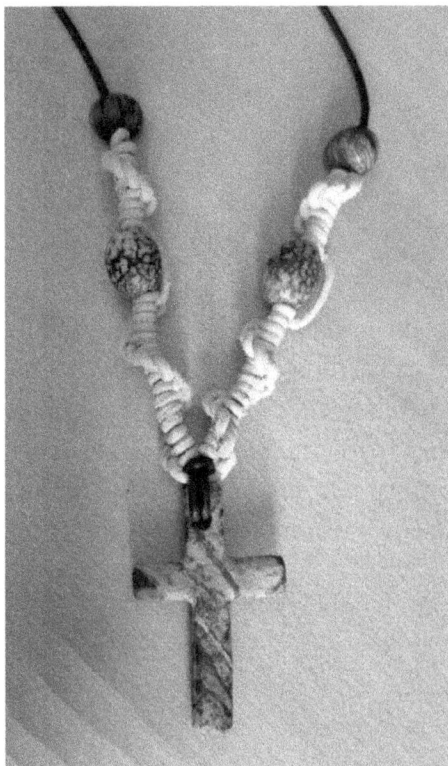

One way to think of the diagnosis, regardless of what name it is given, is as a "wake up call." Once you realize you are here for a reason, you can begin to co-create the life of giving and receiving that God would choose for/with you. This is a critically important time to pay close attention to your "inner voice." These are the messages that come to you when there is a stillness inside you, beyond the voices of fear, anger, worry, or distant memories of the past. Allow for a sense of peacefulness to reside in your heart and mind and welcome the presence of God. When you do this, just be still and listen.

There may be nods of agreement that we each live in an energy field. When we are energetically aligned to our Source/to God, our lives are "in flow" and we feel centered, ready to take on life's enjoyments and challenges. The inner voice messages can feel like a tap on the shoulder to pay attention. If we are "in flow," we notice, and make the small choices and corrections which keep us in alignment with God's choices for/with us.

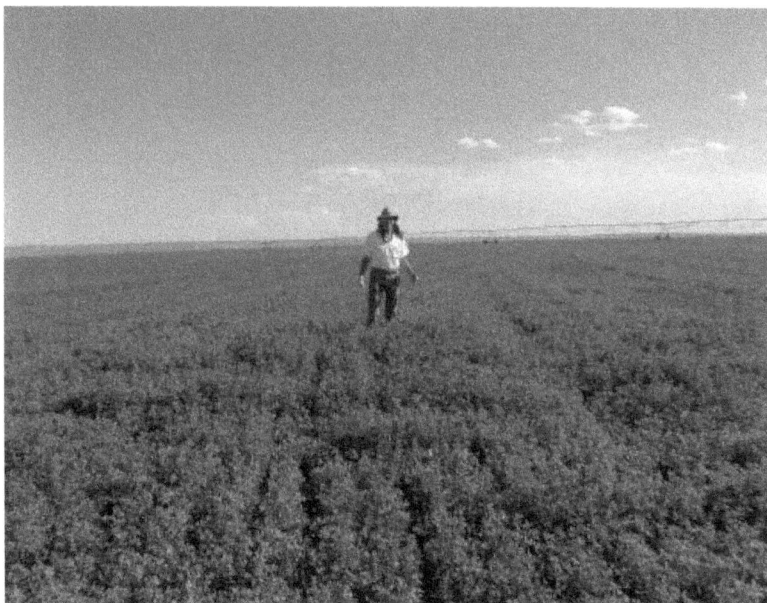

If we choose to ignore the inner guidance, refuse to listen, or pretend we didn't hear, the next level of communication can feel like a thump on the head, then a brick, a truck, and finally a freight train. The art of meditation is an exercise in deep listening. As a daily practice, it can be a powerful resource, along with your familiar religious/spiritual practices.

As you become more and more comfortable listening to your inner guidance, and stepping more fully into your spiritual relationship with God (that is, praying, reading your Bible and/or spiritual literature, selfless service), you will likely discover the thoughts, feelings, words and actions that lead you into confrontation, struggle, and separation from your soul's Highest Good will begin to fall away. The more stressful quality of life, based on behaviors and habits which leave you feeling less than fulfilled, will begin to shift. You may also notice that your attention begins to turn toward what is really wanted and needed to provide more optimal nourishment for your physical, mental, emotional, and spiritual well being.

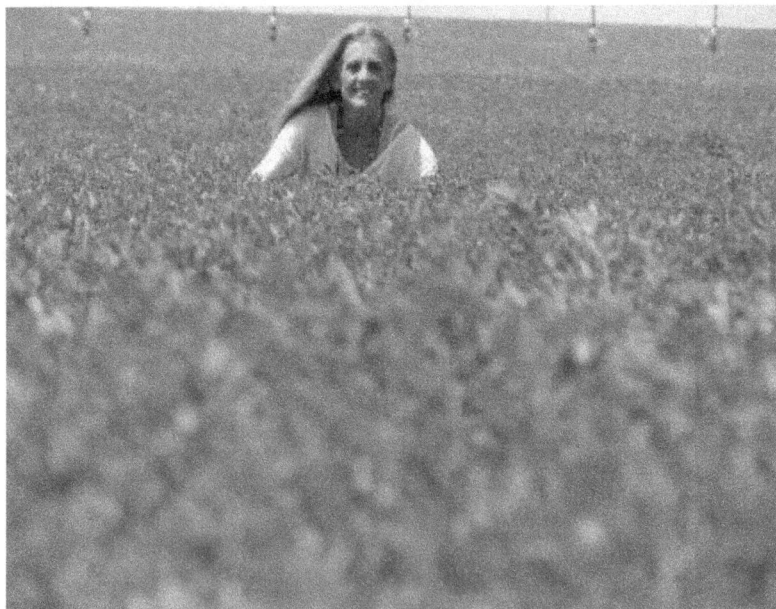

Just remember that, in the weaving of the fabric of your life, there are forces at work which you may call providence, divine intervention, or serendipity. Be willing to allow what you might, in the moment, also call a mistake, or something that feels like a catastrophe, to be recognized as the opening which takes your life in a direction which someday, you will look back on, and refer to as your destiny.

RESOURCES FOR NUTRITION, PHYSICAL EXERCISE, MENTAL & SPIRITUAL ATTUNEMENTS TO LIVING "IN THE POSITIVE"
On-going optimal support to sustain the benefits of The Divine Three Protocol starts with the continuation of using the radiation hormesis stones—the Pendant, Green Stone, Hot Stone, and Mudpack—and the Water Divine Foundation Kit on a daily basis.

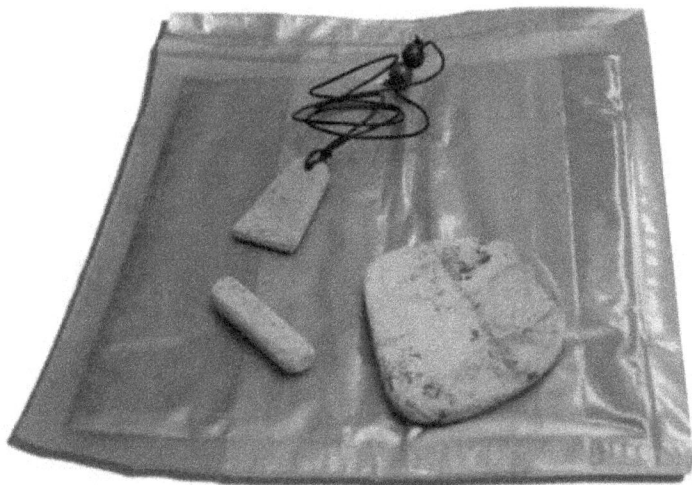

Find the support systems you need for optimal nourishment for your physical, mental, emotional, and spiritual well being. Family, church, a fitness program, courses to advance skills and knowledge, and a circle of friends that give you a strong sense of purpose, connection, and belonging will likely be high priorities.

At Night Hawk Minerals we encourage you to explore possibilities to enrich your life experiences. The few included here are intended to inspire your pursuit of health, happiness, and success in mind, body, and spirit.

1. *The Hormesis Effect: The Miraculous Healing Power of Radioactive Stones*, by Jane G. Goldberg and Jay Gutierrez. Website: SeaRavenPress.com
2. Amazinglifeinstitute.org
3. *Quantum Wellness: A Practical and Spiritual Guide to Health and Happiness*, by Kathy Freston. Website: KathyFreston.com
4. *Gohn Dagow: Movements for Health and Self Defense*, by F. H. Treon. Website: GohnDagow.com
5. *Jesus and the Law of Attraction* and *The Bible and the Law of Attraction*, both by award-winning author Lochlainn Seabrook. Website: SeaRavenPress.com

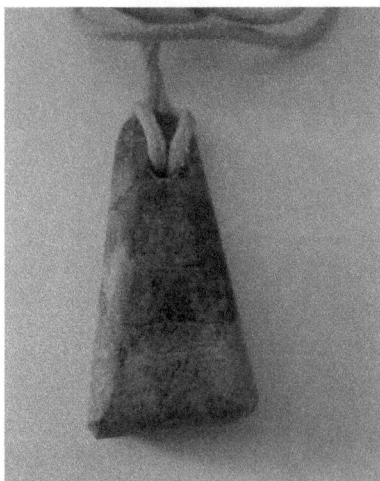

Everything is made up of energy. In the little known martial art book mentioned above (#4), there is a philosophy which states: Just as ripples emanate from a stone tossed into the center of a pond, so good deeds emanate and multiply from us.

This leads to an important question to contemplate for living "in the positive." How will you use your energy to allow the ripples (the frequencies) which flow from your body, mind, and spirit to multiply into ever increasing good deeds and service to fulfill your destiny?

Appendix

NIGHT HAWK MINERALS VOLUNTEER SERVERS PROGRAM

"Even the smallest act of caring for another person is like a drop of water: it will make ripples throughout the entire pond." — Jessy and Bryan Matteo

One of the most important principles for advancing at all levels, both physical and Spiritual, is offering and providing selfless service—the kind of service to others which allows their soul's purpose to be uplifted and soar in the world around them. As this offering becomes a practice in one's life, it deepens the understanding that giving and receiving make a circle of love that knows no difference. This kind of sharing creates an energy field of mutual support which boots out thoughts and feelings of separation, especially fear, and welcomes intentions for unconditional love. In this atmosphere, healing can happen quite rapidly.

It is from this awareness that Night Hawk Minerals offers a Volunteer Servers Program. Here's how it works:

As a person, couple, or family, you become aware of our center in Pritchett, Colorado, and our mission to provide The Divine Three Protocol in the healing process of people with degenerative diseases. You may want to join our Volunteer Servers Program. This can be especially true if one among you is in need of healing, and your desire is to stay for a longer period of time.

You may also want this avenue for the opportunity to discover more about The Divine Three Protocol in this unrecognized field. And, you may want to come because through some divine intervention, you discovered Night Hawk Minerals and simply want to be of service, without personal agenda or thought of reward. However God may have placed Night Hawk Minerals on your radar, all inquiries into the Volunteer Servers Program are welcome.

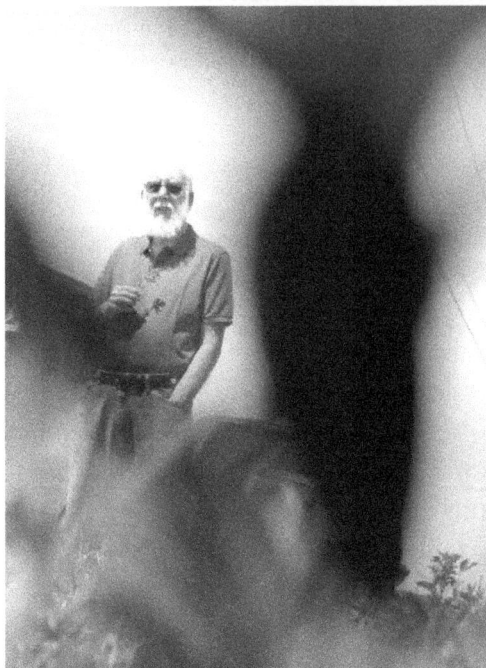

The program is set up for volunteer service to be provided in three hour blocks of time for six hours per day, six days per week. Two hour evening sessions will focus on individual and group processes for nurturing health and well being. Sundays are recognized as personal days for spiritual and religious focus. For volunteers who stay more than two weeks, the third Saturday is a "free day." And for the rest of your tenure, every Saturday and Sunday there after are for your personal choices.

You will be provided with housing in the Rock House or the Golden Quarters of the Volunteer Servers Residence, named the Blue Cottage, two blocks from the Mineral Palace. The Blue Cottage will provide you with internet access, kitchen facilities, and one shared bathroom. Any pets to be considered will have to be discussed and decided upon in each individual situation.

Regarding use of the healing modalities and protocols: a schedule will be set up for your use of the hot stones hot tub and the hot stones frequencies room, as well as ozone sessions in the Mineral Palace. Foot soaks and inhales will be available at the Blue Cottage, as well as essential oil based back, neck, and foot massages. FYI: In a previously designed healing program offered at the Mineral Palace, a seven day program was presented for $5,000.00.

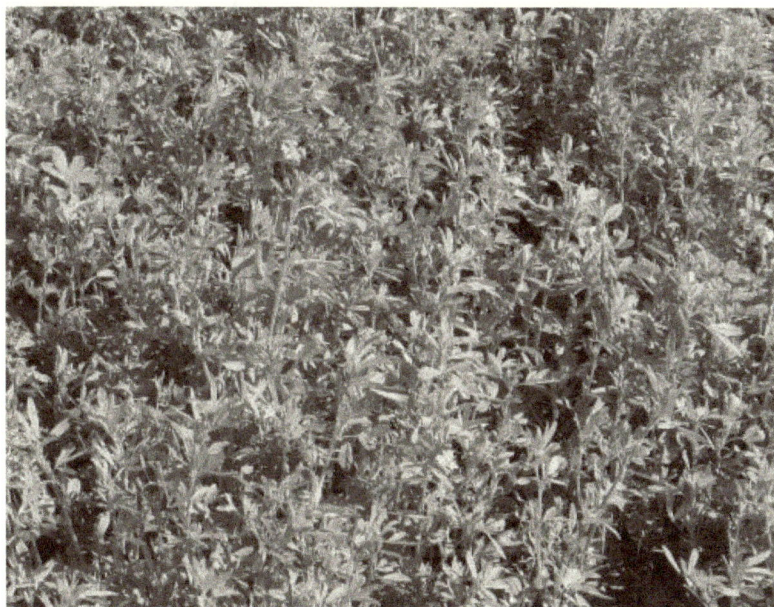

Costs which you must plan to cover include your own use of your personal Pendants, Hot Stones, and Mudpacks; the mineral waters and vitamin packs in the Foundation Kit provided by Water Divine; and the identification and elimination of parasites, including live blood cell analysis and essential oil remedies provided by Dr. d'Angelo and Julia Rose Botanicals.

The total package cost of The Divine Three Protocol, which you would cover, if you choose to support yourself with The Divine Three Protocol, is in the ball park of $1,500.00.

You will also want to be aware of possibilities to offer financial donations. The donations are specifically used to provide protocols for clients needing financial assistance; keeping the Mineral Palace operating at the highest level of support and efficiency; and handling emergencies that would otherwise interfere with the optimal flow of service to clients.

The categories of volunteer service include: personal assistance to the founders of the company; cleaning of the facilities; kitchen and laundry support; grounds keeping; handy man/woman fix it projects; plants and greenhouse attending; and gardening.

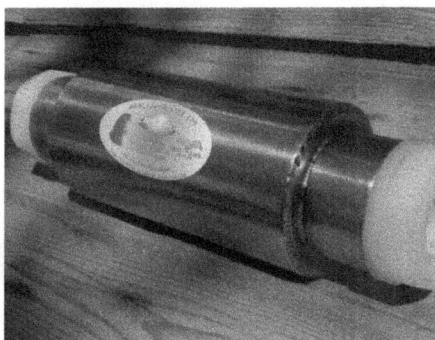

Join Night Hawk Minerals Volunteer Staff Members for one week or longer:

1. Request an application, by email, from Night Hawk Minerals. Contact information is in Section 9. The Volunteer Service Coordinator will send you an application via email. Complete it and return it.

2. If/when the application is accepted, plan for three Skype interviews with the Volunteer Servers Coordinator (VSC) to define your service and prepare for your arrival. We look forward to hearing from you.

THE EXPERIENCE

Over many years now, we here at Night Hawk Minerals have had numerous people make the journey to Pritchett, Colorado, looking for answers on a variety of different challenges. Everything from water to weather, from cattle to cancer, they come here not just for answers, but to witness physical validation and receive personal attention for their particular situation.

The energies that we work with here are for some very hard to grasp and acknowledge until they have been welcomed and can observe for themselves. As far as we know, we are the only ones in the world that work with these kinds of natural technologies. Those that need answers have made this journey. This is why we call this "The Experience."

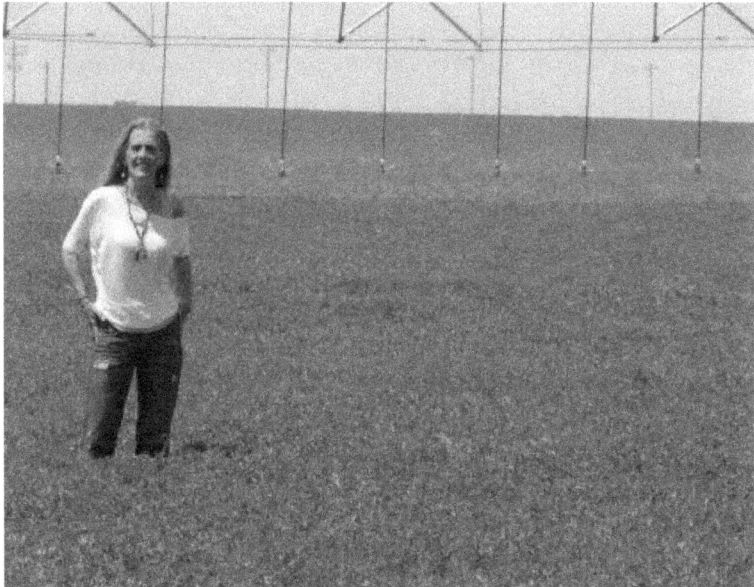

Contact Information

For The Divine Three Protocol and Wellness Instructors

NIGHT HAWK MINERALS (Protocol One)
Mailing Address: PO Box 98, Pritchett, CO 81064 USA
Office telephone: 888-563-8389
Website: NightHawkMinerals.com
Email: info@nighthawkminerals.com
Facebook: facebook.com/Nighthawkminerals
Twitter: twitter.com/healingrocks
Publisher's Website: SeaRavenPress.com

NIGHT HAWK MINERALS WELLNESS INSTRUCTORS
Office telephone: 888-563-8389
Jay Gutierrez: ext. #1
Faye Gutierrez: ext. #2
Daniel Cox: ext. #3
Cisco Sanchez: ext. #6

WATER DIVINE (Protocol Two)
Office telephone: 256-482-2113
Website: WaterDivine.com

PARAWELLNESS RESEARCH (Protocol Three)
Address: 18121 E Hampden Ave Unit C #123, Aurora, CO 80013
Office telephone: 303-680-2288
Website: ParaWellnessResearch.com
Email: drdangelo@parawellnessresearch.com

MEET JAY GUTIERREZ

JAY GUTIERREZ spent 20 years in the Air Force and Army as an F-16 jet engine mechanic and a helicopter engine and airframe mechanic. He has received many awards and has numerous helicopter mission stories.

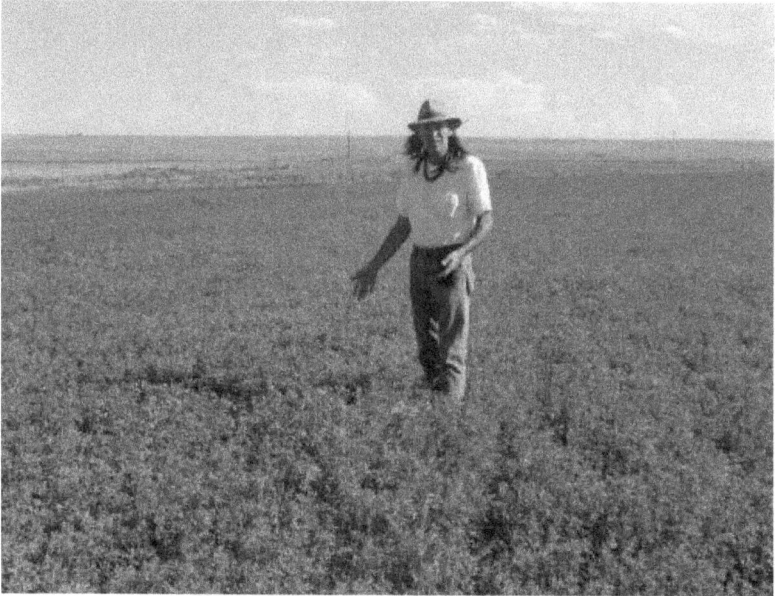

Jay Gutierrez, CEO of Night Hawk Minerals.

One day while flying on a mission he discovered some blue and green stone on the ground and made some jewelry out of it and gave it to some friends. Later he found out the stones were mildly radioactive. He attempted to buy the jewelry back, thinking he may have injured those people he cared about.

Remarkably, instead of their being sick, they remained unusually healthy and attributed that health in large part to wearing those stones. Ever since, Jay has made it his main mission in life to help others become aware of the healing energies associated with low radiation stones.

Today Jay is considered an expert in the field of natural radiation hormesis. After traveling several times around the country and working with clients, doctors, healers, and scientists, he and his wife Faye are now successfully fighting serious degenerative diseases such as cancer. Their company, Night Hawk Minerals, is the only U.S. company they are aware of that actively promotes the use of natural radiation hormesis.

As a byproduct of helping health challenged individuals, Jay has discovered additional ways to use these energies in other important areas affecting all mankind—modalities that he will present in an upcoming book to be published by Sea Raven Press.

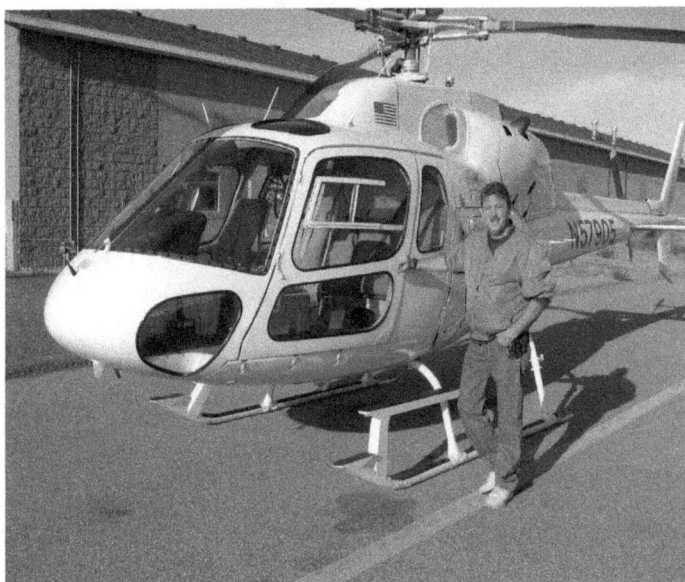

MEET FAYE GUTIERREZ

FAYE GUTIERREZ, co-owner of Night Hawk Minerals, has years of experience as an accomplished Medicine Woman, and is a pioneer in the fields of radiation hormesis and natural frequency medicine.

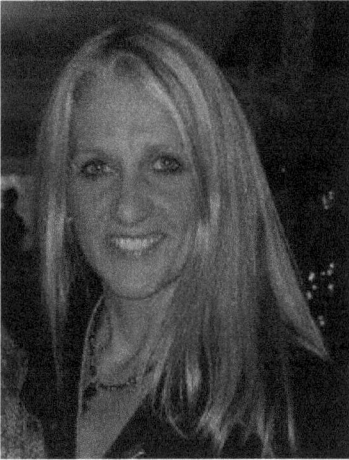

A native of Virginia, Faye is the business negotiator for Night Hawk Minerals, through which she has long successfully helped others suffering from degenerative diseases.

She has also been instrumental in Night Hawk Minerals' many achievements and discoveries, all which are geared toward advancing the health of mankind.

With her vast background, business acumen, and training, she is well-known for her passion, commitment, and fastidious approach to health and healing. Faye continues to positively alter the lives of all those who come in contact with her.

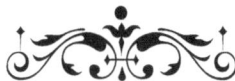

About Night Hawk Minerals

NIGHT HAWK MINERALS offers information and products concerning radiation hormesis, and is headed by founder Jay Gutierrez and Faye Gutierrez.

The Night Hawk Minerals Webstore includes: a full selection of radiation hormesis stones, research material on radiation hormesis, instructions on how to use the stones, articles, PDF files, radio interviews with Jay, FAQ, Jay's video blog, health benefits, information on treating cancer, diabetes, candida, heart problems, general pain issues, autoimmune diseases, and a host of other illnesses, recommended Websites and books, monthly specials, evidence for radiation hormesis, natural living news, testimonials, a history of the company, and Wellness Instructors.

Jay and Faye's books, *The Divine Three Manual: How to Heal Yourself Safely and Simply Using Earth's Natural Resources*, and Jay's book (with Jane G. Goldberg, Ph.D.), *The Hormesis Effect: The Miraculous Healing Power of Radioactive Stones*, are available as paperbacks and ebooks on the Sea Raven Press Webstore.

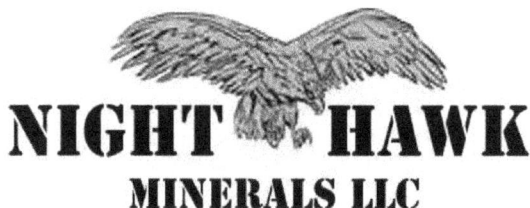

NIGHT HAWK
MINERALS LLC

INDEX

Enjoy our spiritual, mental, and physical health-related titles:

☛ THE HORMESIS EFFECT: THE MIRACULOUS HEALING POWER OF RADIOACTIVE STONES
☛ VITAMIN D: THE MIRACLE TREATMENT FOR NEARLY EVERY DISEASE AND HEALTH ISSUE
☛ VICTORIAN HERNIA CURES: NONSURGICAL SELF-TREATMENT OF INGUINAL HERNIA
☛ JESUS AND THE LAW OF ATTRACTION: THE BIBLE-BASED GUIDE TO CREATING PERFECT HEALTH, WEALTH, AND HAPPINESS FOLLOWING CHRIST'S SIMPLE FORMULA

Available from Sea Raven Press and wherever fine books are sold.

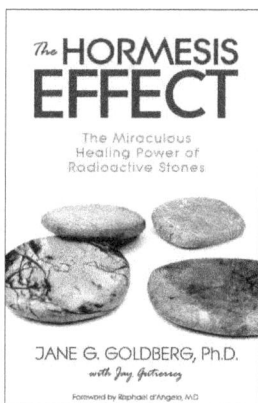

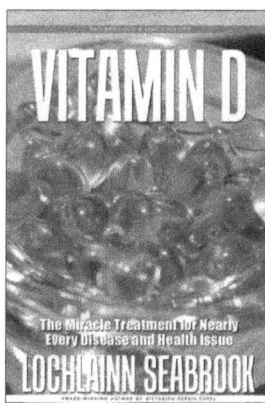

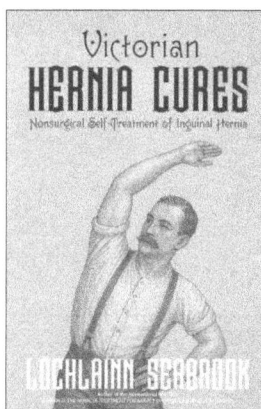

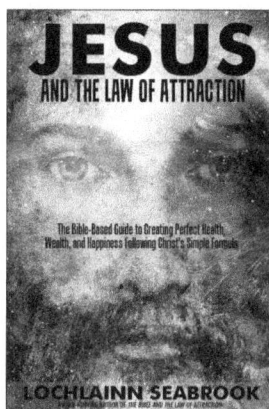

www.ingramcontent.com/pod-product-compliance
Lightning Source LLC
Chambersburg PA
CBHW032353280326
41935CB00008B/561